VOLUME ONE

T. V. Sairam, a senior member of the civil services, holds a Master's degree in botany and a doctorate in alternative medicine. For the past three decades he has been gathering and documenting data relating to the household use of medicinal plants.

Polish Skin Scrub

2 tbsp almond oil
1 heaped tbsp oatmeal } mix
start from ankles and
massage skin.

Face Mask

2 heaped tsp chickpea flour
½ tsp honey
2 tsp water (maybe more)

Apply to face & neck
Leave 15 mins

Home Remedies
Volume One

A Handbook of Herbal Cures for Common Ailments

T. V. SAIRAM

Illustrations by Lena Weyer

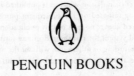

Penguin Books India (P) Ltd, 11 Community Centre, Panchsheel Park, New Delhi-110017, India
Penguin Books Ltd., 27 Wrights Lane, London W8 5TZ, UK
Penguin Putnam Inc., 375 Hudson Street, New York, NY 10014, USA
Penguin Books Australia Ltd., Ringwood, Victoria, Australia
Penguin Books Canada Ltd., 10 Alcorn Avenue, Suite 300, Toronto, Ontario M4V 3B2, Canada
Penguin Books (NZ) Ltd., 182-190 Wairau Road, Auckland 10, New Zealand

First published by Penguin Books India (P) Ltd. 1998

Copyright © T. V. Sairam 1998

Typeset in Adobe Garamond by Eleven Arts. Delhi-35

While every effort has been made to verify the authenticity of the information contained in this book, it is not intended as a substitute for medical consultation with a physician. The publisher and the author are in no way liable for the use of the information contained in the book.

For the innumerable
housewives, ojhas, hakims and vaidyars
who continue to practise their
arts in difficult times

Contents

CONTENTS

Introduction

For cutting off the tender sprouts, a fine of six panas will be imposed; for cutting off the minor branches, twelve panas and for cutting off the big branches, twenty-four panas. Cutting off the trunk will be punished with the first amercement; and felling will be punished with the middlemost amercement.

—Arthashastra, III 19:197

The writing of this book was undertaken to fill what I perceive to be a serious void between the ethnic discovery of herbs and their scientific rediscovery.

It was felt that collecting and categorizing available data from folklore as well as the Western scientific literature on medicinal herbs would facilitate an informed understanding that could better evaluate the premises and methodology of the complicated and often misunderstood role of herbalism and alternative medicine. Herbs are often seen as the last resort once all other avenues of treatment have been exhausted. Being approached as last-minute miracle workers serves to reinforce the mystic aura associated with such systems of medicine, thus discounting the sophisticated and ancient herb lore that its practitioners draw on. The hereditary household remedial system handed down by often unlettered women, the village vaids, hakims and ojhas and their travelling counterparts represent the fragmentary remnants of systems evolved to perfection to meet the needs of localized communities, drawing on familiar plants and locally available materials to treat ailments. Such practices are however fast becoming extinct, and I have often noted on my travels that even in a far-flung village, it has become the fashion to go for a tablet of aspirin rather than a piece of ginger, unmindful of the feeble voice of a family elder or the village physician.

Systematic documentation of this knowledge becomes an urgent necessity in the face of such onslaughts, as has been made clear to me time and again on my frequent trips to remote areas. The Kotas, among one of the ancient inhabitants of the Nilgiris, have all but lost their familiarity with their native medicines. Their villages which till recently boasted of a village physician, now totally depend on the nearby hospitals for treating even the simplest of ailments.

An identical situation prevails in a village near Hyderabad. Almost the entire village was suffering from malnutrition due to vitamin deficiency. The villagers squarely blamed the government for their plight and pointed out that the local dispensaries never maintained adequate stocks of vitamins. All this was in spite of the surprisingly large number of drumstick trees which were growing almost everywhere in the village! All the vitamin-loaded leaves of the trees were ironically ending up as manure or cattle feed.

The ancient methods designed for optimum beneficial use of local resources are in danger in ways that classical systems such as Ayurveda, Unani and Siddha have overcome. These classical systems have been elaborately documented in the form of verses, which survive as manuscripts in the written form, or are passed on from generation to generation orally. Herbal folklore however continues to be unrecorded and as a consequence, endangered.

India has always been a treasure trove of herbs. Historically in traditional Indian cuisine, there was hardly any distinction between food and medicine. Herbs were seen as agents of satisfaction and well being. Centuries before the birth of the

Greek and Roman empires, Indian ships carried herbs and their derivatives like perfumes and textiles to far-off destinations like Arabia, Mesopotamia and Egypt. The subcontinent's wealth of flora derives from the wide variations in geo-climactic and ecological endowments—tropical, temperate, alpine and arid zones, fluctuating factors such as relative humidity, temperature, monsoon, etc. The sheer variety of herbs and spices available to early shamans and physicians and their rich herb mythology and herb lore lured human migration not only from her neighbourhood but also from distant lands.

Later, it was Indian spices that wrote a fascinating history of adventure, exploration, conquest and colonialism. Bitter sea battles were fought over the spice growing colonies. The treasures of herbs and spices have always been indicators of wealth and status and have dictated the policies of nations. Indian herbalism was developed by the ancient seers, sages, wanderers and tribals who through intuition and observation discovered the many properties of plants and their products. The wisdom and experience of generations was consolidated in its growth. Over the millenia, other herbal systems and herbs brought into the subcontinent grew and added to indigenous lore.

Today it is easy to forget that the original sources of modern medicine were unsung folk prescriptions: morphine from poppy, quinine from cinchona, ephedrine from ma-huang, digitalin from foxglove. Today too, there are people who still treat minor ailments inexpensively with remedies taught to them by their forebears. This is especially true of folk medicine and simple home remedies and beauty aids taught to young girls by their grandmothers in many parts of the country. The body of information accumulated in these and other systems of medicine, dealing with the specific medicinal applications of herbs for specific complaints, has been tested innumerable times over the millenia in actual practice.

Scientific Interest in Herbs

The term herb technically refers to a non-woody plant that dies down to the ground after flowering. In general use, it refers to any plant species, including trees. Plants are the chemical factories of nature. The spectacular progress in organic chemistry has rendered most of the natural products amenable to synthesis. In the late eighteenth century and the nineteenth century, organic chemists occupied centre-stage. Recognizing the importance of plant materials, they isolated the active ingredients of many plants and plant products—nimbidin from *Azadirachta indica* (Neem), hyosine from *Datura metel* (Green Thorn Apple), and reserpine from *Rauwolfia serpentina* (Sarpagandha). In the twentieth century, the sixties saw the phytochemists working with randomly chosen plants. In the seventies growing interest in folkloric drugs urged these qualified researchers to select and work on plants used in traditional medicine. In the eighties and nineties these studies, aimed at the isolation and structure elucidation of the chemical constituents of the chosen plants, were pursued further. Despite such investigation, it is estimated that ninety per cent of recorded flora remains unstudied. However, the ultimate aim of scientific interest in traditional drugs is neither to ascribe them formal recognition or to explore their use as just alternatives or supplements to modern medicine.

The medical recipes and therapies gathered by me from diverse sources deserve very serious and urgent consideration by scientific and medical researchers. I think the time has come for the scientific community not to rest content with the isolation of 'active principles' alone from these plants. This 'classical' approach by scientists seeking to pinpoint single active substances and either extract them as they are or synthesize them in the laboratories serves only a limited purpose, since we are already aware that plants also contain secondary enhancing and/or side-effect-eliminating substances, which are lost for good in the process of isolation of active principles. Besides, there is greater scope for researchers to discover which chemical appears in which part of the plant and when. Apart from verifying existing scientific findings and explaining the role of plants in modern biochemical terms, which I understand that the Herb Society in London has currently undertaken, there is a need for a scientific understanding of systems of alternative medicine that have proved useful for suffering humanity, and for which no scientific explanation has yet emerged. The scientific community by transcending its mindset would perhaps be able to find a satisfactory answer to this in the coming years.

Herbalism in India is today beset by myriad problems. The value of the medicinal plant depends on its active principle content and not on its abundant growth or harvest. This aspect distinguishes the herbal industry from the others as the norms of production of agricultural crops differ.

Moreover, it is often found that the same plant grown in different localities differs widely in its medicinal value. Several factors such as soil, rainfall, latitude, altitude, method of cultivation, time of collection, storage, transport, etc play an important role in the medicinal value of drugs.

A wholesome and uniform *Materia Medica* appears a distant dream even today.

What is worse, there is no attempt to identify correct plant species mentioned in various vernacular literatures. There is also no serious attempt to document even today all available information on herbs mentioned in the vernacular treatises lying scattered over the length and breadth of the country, or to confirm and consolidate information relating to the affective part of the plant or its dosage and the application-methodology, particularly the details relating to combining the herbs.

Although most of the vernacular treatises make an attempt to broadly communicate the uses of plants, there is little other detail in them, meant as they are for the expert practising physician. Particulars such as exact dosage, duration of treatment, etc are often left to the imagination of the lay and often unlettered present-day practitioners. There is thus a need for formulating the effective dosage and treatment-duration in respect of each herb/herbal product.

There is also widespread practice of substitution of herbs and ingredients. This is a very serious offence which unfortunately goes unnoticed or un-reported. It is necessary that some institutional checks are initiated with a view to ensure purity and quality of herbal products.

I can find no better way to end, than with this beautiful story that emphasizes the need to preserve our ancient skills. The story tells of the legendary Jivaka, who was the royal physician during Buddha's time.

On completion of his seven-year medical course at Taxila, Jivaka was given the following problem by the examiner: 'Take this spade and seek around Taxila, a yojana on every side and whatever plant you see which is not medicinal, bring it to me.'

Jivaka, so the legend goes, examined all the plants in the specified area and was forced to return to the examiner empty-handed!

How to Use the Book

The book deals with forty commonly found herbs in the subcontinent, most of them familiar kitchen and spice box staples that are invariably accompanied by some minimal knowledge of their therapeutic properties, even in urban homes. The majority of these herbs are indigenous, though some like fenugreek and chillies were brought into the country by incoming invaders, colonisers and migrants. Over a period of time, they have merged so much with Indian gastronomy and medicine that their place of origin appears to be irrelevant. While dealing with each herb, I have recorded its traditional use along with recent scientific information, particularly its efficacy as a drug. A list of references from scientific research work indicating the composition and efficacy of herbs and their constituents will enable each reader to arrive at his or her own evaluation of the relevance of both the traditional practices and the scientific literature. The *In Tradition* pages record the accepted remedies for specific ailments that draw upon each herb's unique therapeutic properties. The ailments are arranged not in alphabetical order, but in groups under the system of related organs to which they belong, as usually classified in medical terminology. They are in their order of presentation in the book, the skeletal and muscular systems (bones, joints, sprains, muscle pulls), the circulatory system (heart, blood, blood vessels, glands, lymph, etc), the digestive system, the excretory system, all fevers and ailments relating to the head, neck and throat, the nervous system, the reproductive system, the respiratory system, the integumentary system (skin, pigmentation, etc) and miscellaneous ailments that do not fall under just one of these heads.

While each entry has been alphabetized, certain groups of related symptoms that cover more than one system have not been separated, since all or a few of them may occur simultaneously. The extensive index at the back of the book allows quick location of multiple remedies for the same ailment, and a choice of herbs. The intuitive preference of certain herbs over others is the best pointer in choosing the appropriate remedy. As many Indian language names as possible have been recorded, thus enabling easy identification of the herbs. The multi language index facilitates the location of herbs by their familiar names, rather than the botanical or English ones. The detailed line drawings that accompany each herb further underline their familiarity while linking us to forgotten healing traditions.

The book records traditional medicinal remedies that are in danger of falling into disuse in forms in which they have been handed down across generations of practitioners. Traditional household practises regarding dosage, application and combination of herbs for alleviating symptoms and curing ailments were all gathered by me mostly through word of mouth from hundreds of housewives, illiterate grandmothers, vaids and ojhas, who voluntarily came forward to reveal them, including specialized tips derived from a lifetime of experience. These living herbals of folk usage will hopefully be the starting points for a comprehensive *Herbal Materia Medica*. Tips on certain herbal preparations that serve as inexpensive substitutes for their chemical-based brethren in the markets are included wherever possible. A comprehensive medical and herbal glossary and one of Non-English terms explains technical concepts from various systems of medicine.

Herbal Preparations: Some Guidelines

There could be some confusion regarding the preparation of home remedies for lay readers. An attempt is made here to explain the various procedures, processes and preparations dealt with in this book.

Notes on Preparation

In traditional systems of medicine, particularly the ones prevalent in South India, one often comes across the practice of mixing honey with almost every herbal powder or *bhasma*, etc. Honey is regarded as an essential vehicle that aids easy digestion and assimilation of the drug. Whenever honey is not available, other sweet substances such as jaggery, sugar candy, etc are powdered and mixed with the drug. As in Ayurveda, balancing of tastes is an important phenomenon and drugs which are bitter, sour or astringent are often mixed with sweet substances and administered.

Resins and Gums. Resins and gums exude from the branches of several trees, especially *Acacia*. They are generally harvested in the dry seasons, by making wounds on their branches and trunks.

The liquid exudate which solidifies quickly is then scraped off the tree with the help of a knife. In the case of myrrh (*Commiphora myrrha*), the exudate is initially pale-yellow in colour, but as it solidifies, it becomes brown-black.

Jams. Herbal jams are solid or semi-solid preparations. The herbal paste or powder is cooked in liquid (water or milk), and ghee, sugar syrup, etc are added while cooking. A jam is ready when it achieves single or double thread consistency and when a dollop sinks into water *en masse* without spreading. A jam made of fresh ginger is a common household remedy used to strengthen the digestive fire, while another made of dry ginger powder is used as a winter tonic. There is a wide variety of jams used therapeutically for indigestion, diarrhoea, piles, bleeding disorders, respiratory problems, reproductive disorders, etc. *Chyavanaprasa,* the most well-known among jams, consists mainly of amla in addition to as many as forty herbs and at times, is fortified with even minerals. It is a rejuvenator and also a remedy for debility and old age.

Medicated Oils and Fats. Sneha are prepared by boiling a drug-fat-water mixture until the water evaporates and the remnants are strained. There are four textures distinguishable in Kerala preparations: flowing, soft, waxy and hard. While hair oils (often medicated with amla, Chinese rose, etc) are flowing, certain preparations like medicated ghee are in various semi-solid states (soft, waxy or hard). Soft fats are used for nasal medication. Waxy fats are used for internal consumption and the hard greasy ones are applied to the body. The hard fat often contains charred herbs.

Nasal and Eye Drops. Nasal and eye medication is preferred for purification in all diseases of the head, lungs, throat and eyes. A good daily routine includes introduction of a couple of drops of medicated oil or ghee into the nose or eyes as the case may be. Whenever any fresh juice is required to be introduced, sufficient caution is to be exercised to avoid any contamination.

Sterilized cotton and clean hands are necessary. Never use more than 2–3 drops at a time.

Application of Warmed Leaves. Some leaves are applied on boils, etc after warming over a flame. The leaves which are otherwise hard or leathery get softened and pliable by such treatment and are rendered handy for bandaging the affected area. Sometimes a coating of oil (such as sesame oil) is applied on the surface of the leaves before warming them.

Burning the Plant Materials. This process is quite common and releases the aroma (e.g., resins, incense, etc) of the plant parts which helps in relieving nasal congestion, etc. In certain cases, plant parts are burnt over hot coals and the ash obtained is used as medicine.

Roasting the Plant Materials. Roasting plant parts such as seeds is a common method before they are used as medicine. By roasting in the skillet, the volatile oil content in seeds is gradually released and the efficacy of the plant parts, when used as medicine, increases. In Siddha medicine, roasting of leaves, etc is also done in mud pots. Such a roasting process removes traces of moisture, besides wilting the leaves.

A Note on Dosage

> *A doctor should treat taking account of the patient,*
> *the illness and the time.*
>
> —Tirukkural 949

Prescribing the optimal dosage of the plant material for a particular ailment and for the particular constitution of the patient has always been quite a challenging task for any herbalist. The main reason for this is the fact that the content of the so-called 'active principle' of a plant part varies widely due to factors such as climate, altitude, latitude, soil type, nutrition, temperature, relative humidity, season, time of plucking, packing, storage, etc. Determining the nature of the constitution of the patient has also been a crucial factor for determining the dosage of the drug.

As such, the dosage should vary from person to person and from drug to drug, the judgement being based on the close observation by the physician of the individual constitution and reaction of the patient, with a view to enhance or decrease the dose already prescribed by him. In other words, a close rapport between the physician and the patient is a *sine qua non* before making any such attempt. The practitioner should be fully aware of the inherent weakness in prescribing the dosage, or a particular dose of a drug, in a general or casual way, overlooking the importance of both the dynamism that a drug exhibits and the individuality of a patient's constitution. The crude manner in which dosage has been prescribed in this book is merely to broadly document roughly how much of the drug could be required. It has been assumed that the patient is fully grown and mature. The dosage indicated is therefore subject to modification by the prudent user.

Finally, I make no apologies for the fact that I approach patients like a 'primitive' shaman. For me, they represent highly complex psycho-physico-spiritual creatures rather than mechanical devices, taken up for servicing or repair. I am fully convinced that when a man suffers from an ailment, all he needs is relief best suited to his bodily constitution and in the least harmful way. It is in such a spirit that I hope readers too will approach the book.

Notes on Preparing Plant Parts

Collection. Although there are no hard and fast rules, the following principles are generally adhered to:

Roots, Rhizomes and Bark: They are collected in late autumn or early spring when vegetative growth has ceased.

Leaves and Flowering Tops: They are collected at the time of development of flowers and before maturing of fruit and seed as the photosynthetic activities are maximum at this time. The active principle content is also high.

Fruits: They are collected when fully grown, but unripe.

Seeds: They are collected when fully matured and if possible, before the fruits open for dispersal. Seed-like fruits such as coriander, saunf, ajwain, etc are harvested a little before they are fully ripe, to retain their fresh and bright appearance.

Drying: The object of drying is to remove moisture and to preserve the plant and its parts. Under natural conditions, the drug could be dried under the sun or in shade, according to the nature of its content or the active principle. Greater success is encountered in commercial drying, where the temperature and flow of air are controlled. Certain delicate drugs such as digitalis need a specific temperature for drying.

Garbling: The final stage in the processing of a drug is garbling. In this process, extraneous matter such as dirt, unwanted plant parts, adulterants, etc, are removed.

Packing: Different drugs need different types of packing. Basically, packing should ensure protection against moisture, fungus, insects, etc.

Storage and Preservation: Conditions for storage and preservation vary from plant to plant. In case of drugs such as digitalis, which deteriorate in the presence of moisture, the insertion of a suitable dehydrating substance in the container itself is a prerequisite. In general, the ideal conditions for preservation of all drugs are refrigeration or low temperatures.

Infusion: An infusion, like tea, is made by combining boiling water with herbs (usually the green parts or flowers) and steeping for 5 to 10 minutes to extract their active ingredients. Due to exposure to heat only for a short duration, this method ensures that the volatile elements and vitamins are not totally lost. It is recommended that a porcelain, enamel or glass pot be used while steeping the herbs. The pot should be covered with a tight-fitting lid to minimize evaporation. Sometimes sugar or honey can be added to the infusion to improve its taste. Most herb-teas (also called tisanes) are taken in small regular doses ranging from a teaspoon to a mouthful over a period of time. They are taken quite hot, if the intention is to break up a cold or cough. Otherwise they can be taken either lukewarm or cold.

Decoction: Hard materials such as wood-pieces, bark, roots, seeds, etc require prolonged boiling to extract their active ingredients. About $1/2$ cup of plant parts can be boiled in 1 cup water. It is better to use a non-metallic or enamelled pot. Green plant parts and flowers can be added to cold water, brought to a boil and allowed to remain so for 3–4 minutes. Or they can be added straight to boiling water and allowed to be immersed at a galloping boil for a few minutes. In either case the pot should be covered with a lid. Harder materials need to be boiled longer. Plant parts need to be strained out from the decoction. The Kerala physicians often strain the decoction and boil it again until it is reduced to one-and-a-half times the original weight of the herbs. For cooking decoctions clay pots are considered the best. However, copper pots for *kapha* problems, silver or bronze for *pitta* problems and gold or iron pot for *vata* problems are also considered acceptable and good.

Cold Extract: To ensure effective extraction of delicate or volatile compounds the herbs are steeped in a non-metallic or enamelled pot containing cold water (1:6 ratio of herb and water) for 8 to 12 hours. Strain and the drink is ready. Through this method, only minor amounts of mineral salts and bitter principles can be extracted. Compared to hot infusions, cold extracts would need double the quantity of plant material. This method is recommended for very delicate herbs such as hibiscus, sandalwood, jasmine, marigold, rose, coriander, vetiver, etc and for the treatment of *pitta* conditions.

Juice: While extracting juice from the plant material, a little cold water could be added. This is a good method for extracting water-soluble constituents, vitamins and minerals from the plant.

The juice should be consumed immediately after pressing, as otherwise the vitamin content is denatured and the fermentation process starts. This method is used in the case of all juicy plants particularly aloe, amlaki, brahmi, coriander, garlic, ginger, tulsi, lime, neem, onion, etc.

Syrup: The plant materials can be boiled in honey and strained through cheesecloth. This is an easier way of administering medicines to children.

Powder: Dried plant parts can be ground with the help of a traditional mortar and pestle or with a grinder or blender. Powders made from a combination of a number of drugs are popular in Ayurveda. The versatile *Triphala* is a shining example. The powder can be taken with water, milk or soup. It can be just swallowed with water or sprinkled on food. The common dosage is stated as the quantity that you can lift on the tip of a dinner-knife! These days, gelatine capsules can be used to facilitate swallowing. Sometimes powders are used externally as in the case of *Dashanga Lepa*, which contains liquorice, valerian, red sandalwood, cardamom, turmeric, etc. It is dusted on boils, mumps, abscesses, erysipelas and neuralgia.

Poultice: Also called cataplasm, the poultice is used to apply a herbal product to a skin area with moist heat. Often, the herb is made into a pulpy mass and warmed up. The warmed pulp is spread on a wet, hot cloth and wrapped around the affected area. In the case of mustard pulp or similar herbs, which are quite irritable to the skin, two layers of cloth could be used. After removing the poultice, the area could be washed with water or herbal tea to wipe out any left-over residue on the skin. Poultices are used to soothe, to irritate, or to draw out impurities from the body. Such an action depends on the type of herb selected for the purpose.

Fomentation: A Turkish towel can be soaked in a hot infusion or decoction and after wringing out the excess liquid, applied as hot as possible on the affected area.

Cold Compress: It is like fomentation, but the infusion or decoction used is cold. The cloth is left on the body until it is warmed by body heat. Usually it is left on for 10 to 15 minutes. This is repeated with another fresh cold compress.

Soap Substitutes. Certain plants contain a compound called saponin, which produces lather when the plant tissues are rubbed in water. They can also be used to make shampoos. The plants which contain saponin in sufficient quantity to produce lather are:

Papaya leaves

Soap-nut powder (reetha) and shikakai

Powder made of dried orange rind, lemon rind, rose petals, etc. All these can play an effective role as a substitute for soap.

Turmeric powder, which is a germicide, is also used along with besan, *kasturi manjal,* etc. Powdered leaves of neem, curry-leaf, etc also find their use in substituting soap.

In combination with milk, these herbs make an ideal wash for the upkeep of skin and in preventing its damage due to weather, old age, bacteria, etc.

Volatile Oils: Volatile oils extracted from various plants have been in use from time immemorial. They are extracted by distilling grass (*Cymbopogon,* etc), leaves (basil, cinnamon, *Citrus,* etc), flowers (*Citrus,* jasmine, rose, saffron, etc), flower buds (lawsonia, mango, etc) fruits (black pepper, bel, cardamom, nutmeg, etc), seeds (anise, ajwain, coriander, cumin, saunf, etc), roots or rhizomes (galangal, ginger, sweet flag, turmeric, vetiver, etc), wood (agar, camphor, deodar, sandal, etc), bark (asafoetida, *boswellia,* camphor, commiphora, etc.)

The volatile oils are responsible for the characteristic odour of the plant. Some act on the Central Nervous System, increase appetite, aid digestion and regularize intestinal action. When placed on intact skin, they can increase the flow of blood, especially of leucocytes. This property associated with the bactericidal properties of certain oils is the basis of their antiseptic use.

1

Bel
Aegle marmelos

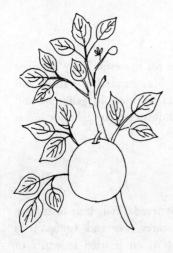

Plant a bel and please Shiva.

—Padma Purana

Bestower of Kingdoms

The orthodox Hindus circumambulate the bilva or bel tree before they attempt any new venture as it is considered to be a tree auspicious to Lord Shiva and Lakshmi, the Goddess of Wealth. It is believed that success in the venture will be assured by doing so.

There is a legendary tale of Vasuman, the king of the Videhas, who is said to have regained his lost kingdom by circumambulating the bel tree in the temple at Tiruvidaimaruthur.

The tree is native to India. The Yajur Veda makes a reference to bel fruit. *Charaka Samhita* recognizes its medicinal potential.

The Root

In Bastar, the tribals use the infusion of roots in the treatment of toxic fevers. The ancient Ayurvedic texts also prescribe the roots as a good restorative tonic. The bel root forms one of the ten precious ingredients of the group of *dasmoolah* (ten-roots), a most popular formulation. The anti-bacterial potentiality of the bel root has been confirmed recently.

The Leaves

The leaves make excellent poultices for the eyes. They are used to cure ulcers, hypertension, jaundice, headache, nausea and *pitta*-aggravations. They are used as poultices in gangrene and inflammations. The leaf juice is administered to diabetics and is found to cure both colds and fever.

The Unripe Fruit

The unripe fruit finds its use in Ayurveda. It is hot, unctuous, intense, stimulates digestion and cures *vata* and *kapha*. It is made into a medicinal jam (*leha*) which is used in acute or chronic diarrhoea, especially where there is alternating diarrhoea and constipation. It is also useful in soothing ulceration of the intestines.

The Ripe Fruit

The ripe fruit is heavy and not easily digested. It is usually made into a cooling astringent sherbet. It is a laxative and tends to disturb the *doshas*. However, it has certain valuable wound-healing tannins which coat the stomach mucosa with mucilage, thus protecting the whole region from possible damage by the fiery stomach-acid. It is therefore recommended to patients suffering from stomach ulcer. In Cambodia, it is used for treating TB and hepatitis.

The Profile

Botanical Names	:	*Aegle marmelos* (Corr.) *Crataeva marmelos* L.
English Names	:	Bel, Bengal Quince, Wood Apple, Golden Apple.
Indian Names	:	Assamese, Bengali, Hindi & Marathi : *Bel* Gujarati : *Bili* Kannada : *Bil Patre* Malayalam & Tamil : *Vilvam* Oriya : *Bilva, Sriphal* Telugu : *Muredu*
Family	:	Rutaceae.
Appearance	:	Thorny tree with edible ripe fruits. Leaves are trifoliate. Flowers greenish-white, sweet-scented and in small bunches. Fruit, large and round with greenish-grey woody shell. Pulp inside is orange in colour with many seeds covered with fibrous hairs, aromatic.
Distribution	:	Occurs in plains almost throughout India. Also reported in Baluchistan, Burma, China and Sri Lanka.
Medicinal Parts	:	Root, bark, leaves, flowers and fruits.

3

In Tradition

AILMENT	PRESCRIPTION
✤ High blood pressure	: Finely powder dried bel leaves and store in a jar. Dissolve $1/2$ to 1 tsp of this powder in 1 teacup water and boil. Cool and filter and drink thrice a day.
✤ Jaundice	: Finely grind some bel leaves. Take 1 tsp of this paste along with a pinch of black pepper and follow with 1 teacup buttermilk thrice a day.
✤ Appetite loss	: Clean some leaves and grind into a paste. Take $1/2$ tsp every morning for 3 days.
✤ Constipation, dyspepsia, mouth ulcer	: Mix the pulp of a ripe fruit with jaggery and eat once a day.
✤ Diarrhoea	: Slice the tender unripe fruits. Sun dry them. Powder. Take 1 tsp along with warm water twice a day.
✤ Diarrhoea, digestive disorders, ulcer	: Take a small, tender budding fruit and grind it with 1 tbsp curd. Take 1 to 2 tsp.
✤ Stomach disorders, glandular enlargement in abdomen, peptic ulcer, fever	: Soak 2 or 3 bel leaves in 1 teacup water. Keep in a copper vessel overnight and drink the water early next morning. Continue for 40 days.

❧ Dysentery : Take 1 teacup fruit pulp twice a day (if mixed with jaggery it can be taken 3 times a day).

❧ Ulcer in mouth/ stomach : Mix 1 teacup pulp with 1 tsp sugar and eat early morning on an empty stomach for 3 days.

❧ Ulcer in stomach : Soak 2 or 3 bel leaves in 1 teacup water overnight and drink the water early next morning.

❧ Piles : Take an unripe fruit and pound it along with 1 tsp each dried ginger and saunf and soak these in 4 teacups water. Sip this water 3 to 4 times a day.

❧ Fever, malaria : Extract 1 tsp each juice from tulsi leaves and bel flowers. Add 1 tsp honey. Take twice a day.

❧ Eye disease, redness in eyes : Pluck a handful of tender leaf buds and roast in a mud pot. Tie them in a muslin cloth and apply on eyelids, when bearably warm.

❧ Watery sperm : Soak 1/4 tsp bel gum in a glass of water overnight. Drink the water early next morning.

❧ Excessive bleeding during menstruation : Grind some leaves into a fine paste. Take 1 tsp with warm water and drink some cold water as well. (*Note*: One has to include milk and curd and avoid chillies and tamarind during this treatment.)

❧ Early stages of
  TB

: Mix the pulp of the ripe fruit with required quantity of sugar and honey and take after dinner for 40 days.

❧ Asthma

: Chew a bel leaf along with 3 or 4 black peppercorns early in the morning. 1 teacup warm milk can also be taken. Continue for 30–40 days.

❧ Pox, smallpox

: Mix 1 tbsp pulp of the ripe fruit (after removing fibres and seeds) in 1 teacup cow's milk (boiled and cooled) and drink.

❧ Body weakness

: Mix 1 tbsp pulp of ripe fruit with 1 tsp palmyrah candy (or sugar) and eat frequently.

❧ Body heat,
  burning eyes

: Take a tender fruit. Grind it in 1 teacup milk. Apply on head and massage well before showering off.

❧ Body heat,
  headache, nausea,
  vomiting

: Pluck a handful of bel leaves and roast in a mud pot. Add 1 teacup water and allow it to boil well. Remove from fire and filter. Take half of it in the morning and the remaining half in the evening. Continue for 21 days. (*Note*: If desired, a little sugar can be added.)

❧ Body weakness, burning sensation in eyes, headache, body heat, diseases of the brain

: Take 3 tbsp each of the following: fruit-pulp of bel, babchi (*Psoralea coryllifolia*) and fenugreek. Add 1 teacup milk and grind into a fine paste. Add this to 2 teacups gingelly oil and boil thoroughly. Cool, filter and store it in a bottle. Apply this oil on the head and massage well before a shower.

Note: Individual results may vary.

A Word of Caution

Excess intake of bel pulp produces atony of the intestine causing flatulence and a sensation of heaviness.

Bel pulp should be chewed thoroughly and it should not be gulped down. If taken hurriedly, it may cause a sensation of heaviness.

In Science

Banerji, N. and R. Kumar. 1980. Studies on the seed-oil of *Aegle marmelos* and its effect on some bacterial species. *J. Inst. Chem. India* 52:59. (Bel's bactericidal seed-oil.)

Banerji, N. et al. 1982. Pharmacognosy of *Aegle marmelos* (L) Correa. Seeds: A new protein source. *Acta Pharma Hung.* 52:97. (Nutritional value of seeds of bel.)

Bhatt, R. M. V. and U. K. Mukul. 1984. Study of *Dashmul*—antibacterial activity. *J. Nat. Integ. Med. Assoc.* 26 (11):319–322. (Bel roots' germicidal properties.)

Chakraborty, T. and G. Poddar. 1984. Herbal drug in diabetes, Part I. Hypoglycaemic activities of indigenous plants in streptozotocin induced diabetes in rats. *J. Inst. Chem. India* 56 (Part I):20–22. (Bel's use in diabetes.)

Dhar, M. L. et al. 1968. Screening of Indian plants for biological activity, Part-I. *Indian J. Exptl. Biol.* 6:232. (Bel fruit's efficiency against the Ranikhet virus.)

Harvey, S. K. 1968. A preliminary communication of the action of *Aegle marmelos* (Bel) on heart. *Indian J. Med. Res.* 56:327. (Bel leaves' cardiac stimulant action on frogs' hearts comparable with that of digitoxin, the well-known drug.)

Jain, S. K. and C. R. Tarafdar. 1970. Medicinal plant-lore of the Santals. *Econ. Bot.* 24(3):241–278. (Bel as a cure for snake-bites.)

Kakiuchi, N. et al. 1990. Effects of constituents of bel (*Aegle marmelos*) on spontaneous beating and calcium only paradox (sic) of myocardial cells. *Plant. Med.* 57(1):43–46. (A study.)

Karunanayake, E. H. et al. 1984. Oral hypoglycaemic activity of some medicinal plants of Sri Lanka *J. Ethnopharmacol.* 11(2):223–231. (Bel as a cure for diabetes.)

Lamba, B. V. and K. P. Bhargava. 1969. Activity of some synthetic and natural products against experimental Ankylostomiasis. *Indian J. Pharmac.* 6. (The bel fruits' use against hookworms.)

Mhaskar, K. S. and J. F. Cains. 1931. Indian plant remedies used in snake-bite. *Indian Med. Res. Mem.* 19:12. (Bel cures snake-bites.)

Ponnachan, P. T. et al. 1993. Hypoglyaemic effects of alkaloids of preparations from leaves of *Aegle marmelos. Amala Res. Bull.* 13(August):37–39. (Bel can bring down the sugar-level.)

Prakash, A. and S. Prasad. 1969. Pharmacognostical studies on the bark of *Aegle marmelos* Correa. *Jour. Res. Ind. Med.* 4(1):97. (Medicinal value of the bark, root and stem.)

Vyas, D. S. et al. 1979. Preliminary study on anti-diabetic properties of *Aegle marmelos* and *Enicostemma littorale. Jour. Res. Ind. Med. Yoga & Homoeo.* 14:3. (Diabetes can be cured by the bark.)

2

Onion

Allium cepa

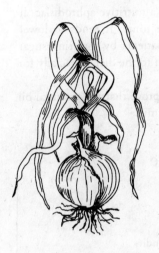

There is no substance which is absolutely of good or bad qualities. Hence our concern should be to select such substances as possess more of the required good qualities.

—Charaka

The Oldest Cultivated Herb

Onion is considered the oldest cultivated herb. For the ancient Egyptians, onion was both food and medicine.

The ancient sages of India, Atreya and Dhanvantri, had acknowledged the utility of the onion in fighting ailments.

Onion in Gastronomy and in Medicine

Onion has a universal appeal in gastronomy. Besides its bulbs, its green shoots, flowers and seeds—all have found their way into the kitchen. Incidentally, all these parts are also reputed to possess certain medicinal uses traditionally in households in India.

Due to the presence of several sulphur compounds, freshly expressed onion juice is found to possess moderate bactericidal properties. As an antiseptic, onion helps to end putrefactive and fermentative processes in the gastro-intestinal tract. Modern research laboratories have recorded the definite anti-tumour activity of onion.

Raw onion is traditionally used as a nutritive aphrodisiac. It is a stimulant as well as a restorative tonic. It tends to lower blood pressure and benefit diabetic patients by lowering sugar levels. It is like garlic, an ideal addition to the diet, especially for those who consume high-fat food.

There is experimental evidence to prove that the essential oil found in onion prevents hyperlipidaemia.

The Profile

Botanical Name	:	*Allium cepa* L.	
English Name	:	Onion.	
Indian Names	:	Assamese, Hindi, Punjabi, Urdu & Bengali	: *Piyaz*
		Gujarati	: *Dunzari*
		Kannada & Telugu	: *Nirulli*
		Kashmiri	: *Kankani, Kandu*
		Konkani	: *Kandu*
		Marathi	: *Kanda*
		Sanskrit	: *Palandu*
		Sindhi	: *Dungari*
		Tamil	: *Vengayam*
Family	:	Liliaceae.	

Appearance	:	The plant consists of a prominent bulb, formed by the thickening of the leaf-base when mature. Leaves are long, linear and hollow. Florets are white.
Distribution	:	All over India.
Medicinal Parts	:	Bulb, shoots, flowers, seeds.
Preparation and Dosage	:	*Juice*: 1 tsp 3 or 4 times a day. *Cold Extract*: Soak a chopped onion in 1 teacup water for 24 hrs. *Dosage*: $1/2$ teacup a day, after straining. *Decoction*: Boil a chopped onion in 1 teacup water. *Dosage*: 1 tbsp taken many times a day.

In Tradition

AILMENT	PRESCRIPTION
❦ Pain in limbs due to arthritis	: Mix equal quantities of onion juice with warm mustard oil and apply on the affected parts.
❦ Cholesterol, thickening of the arterial walls	: Finely dice an onion and mix it with 1 cup buttermilk along with $1/4$ tsp pepper powder and drink.
❦ Stomach ache, hoarseness, cough	: Take 1 tsp onion juice mixed with 1 tsp honey.
❦ Stomach ache, indigestion	: Crush an equal quantity of onions and onion flowers and extract 1 tsp juice. Add 1 tsp honey and drink twice a day.

11

- Ear diseases, certain types of deafness
: Raw onion juice as ear drops.

- Eyesight improvement
: Juice of onion flowers, used as eye drops.

- Gum diseases, toothache
: Crush equal quantities of onions and onion flowers and extract the juice. Gargle frequently with this.

- Headache
: Crush an onion and apply the paste on the head.

- Sexual debility, weakness
: Onion seeds dried and powdered, 1 tsp eaten 3 times daily along with sugar or honey.

- Venereal diseases
: Boil 1 teacup white onions in 2 teacups cow's milk till the milk is thickened. Remove from the fire and add 1 tbsp sugar, 1 teacup wheat flour and 2 teacups ghee and mix the ingredients well till a jam-like consistency is reached. Bottle. *Dosage:* 1 tbsp thrice daily. (*Note:* If excess urination is noticed, then this medicine can be taken on alternate days.)

- Dry coughs
: Mix and fry in 1 tsp ghee 1 tsp each onions and onion flowers. Add 1 tsp jaggery and eat.

- Abscess/pustule
: Cook an onion in olive oil and cover

the abscess or pustule for the discharge of pus.

🌿 Boils : Roast an onion over a naked fire. Pulp to be applied on affected parts, when cooled.

🌿 Suppurating wounds : Apply onion juice on the affected parts.

🌿 Whitlow : Blend together 1 tbsp cooked rice, 1 onion and a little salt. Apply the paste on the affected finger and bandage it.

: Roast a big onion over a naked flame and mash it. Mix in 1 tsp each turmeric powder and ghee and apply on the affected area and tie a bandage.

🌿 Water accumulation in limbs, etc : Boil a few onions in 4 teacups water. Add salt to taste and drink frequently.

🌿 Unconsciousness due to giddiness : Raw onion juice used as nasal drops.

🌿 Toxicity caused by tobacco : Take 1 tsp onion juice.

🌿 Shock : Inhale fresh crushed onions.

🌿 Piles, psoriasis, *pitta*-aggravation : Very thin slices of onions fried in ghee, eaten frequently. (*Caution*: Excess intake may cause coughing and gas in stomach.)

❧ Piles,   : Sliced onion shoots fried in ghee and
constipation,   eaten frequently. (*Caution*: This should
stomach ache,   not be given to children continuously.)
eyesight
problems

Note: Individual results may vary.

A Word of Caution

Excess intake of onion is reported to cause coughing or flatulence.

In Science

Augusti, K. T. 1996. Therapeutic value of onion (*Allium cepa* L.) and garlic (*Allium sativum* L.). *Indian J. Exp. Bio.* 34, 7:634–640. (Onion's therapeutic role.)

Bandyopadhyay, G. et al. 1973. Comparative studies on some chemical aspects of white and red globe onions. *J. Fd. Sci. Technol.* 10(4):169–172. (Chemical affinities and differences between red and white varieties.)

Bhushan, S. et al. 1984. Effect of oral administration of raw onion on glucose tolerance test of diabetics—a comparison with tolbutamide. *Curr. Med. Pract.* 28(12). (Onions in the diet reduced the required dose of anti-diabetic drugs and produced beneficial results in diabetic patients.)

Chopra, R. N. et al. 1956. *Glossary of Indian Medicinal Plants.* New Delhi: Council of Scientific and Industrial Research. (The anti-tumour activity of onions.)

Gupta, R. K. et al. 1977. Blood sugar lowering effect of various fractions of onion. *Indian J. Exptl. Biol.* 15(4):313–314. (Onions lower blood sugar levels.)

Handa, G. et al. 1982. Antiasthmatic principles of *Allium cepa*. *Indian Drugs* 20:239. (How onion combats asthma.)

Nerkar, D. P. et al. 1981. Cytotoxic effect of onion extract on mouse fibro-sarcoma 180A cells. *Indian J. Exptl. Biol.* 19(7):598–600. (Onion extract fights cancer.)

Sharma, K. K. et al. 1975. Studies on hypocholestraemic activity of onion (1) experimentally induced and consequently decreased fibrinolytic activity in rabbits (2) Effect on serum cholesterol in alimentary lipaemia in man. *Indian J. Med. Res.* 63(11):1629–1634. (Onion juice can bring down cholesterol levels.)

Sharma, K. K. et al. 1977. Antihyperglycaemic effect of onion. Effect on fasting blood sugar and induced hyperglycaemia in man. *Indian J. Med. Res.* 65(3):422–429. (Onion juice can lower blood sugar levels.)

Singhvi, S. et al. 1984. Effect of oral administration of onion and garlic on blood lipids. *Rajasthan Med. J.* 23(1):3–6. (In spite of high fat diets, essential oils of onion and garlic prevent the hyperlipidaemic state and act as antidotes in patients prone to hyperlipidemia.)

3

Garlic

Allium sativum

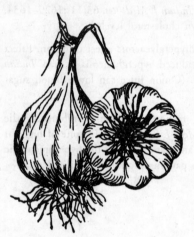

It is ordered that all my workers take garlic every day to maintain their health and strength.

—Khnoom Khoufouf
The Builder of the Ancient Pyramids (4500 B.C.)

Garlic in Traditional Medicine

Ayurveda prescribes six essential tastes which help in balancing *dosha*-aggravation. Of these, garlic exhibits five with the sole exception of the sour taste: pungency resides in its bulb, bitterness in the leaves, salinity at the crown, astringency in the stem and sweetness in the seeds.

Garlic has been held in high esteem for its medicinal use for over six thousand years.

It is considered a powerful rejuvenative herb. It is an effective detoxifier as it cleanses blood and lymph. It tends to dilate peripheral blood vessels and as a result, the blood pressure is lowered. It acts as a stimulant and antibiotic.

Topically, the fresh juice of garlic is effective for acne and other skin infections. Internally, fungal infections, chest problems, digestive disorders and the risk of thromboses are all controlled by regular garlic intake.

The Oil

Garlic derives its peculiar smell from its sulphur-containing volatile oil which accounts for most of its medicinal properties. The oil has an antibiotic action on the gastro-intestinal tract. It spreads throughout the body and is secreted along with toxic wastes, via sweat, urine, faeces, etc.

The bactericidal effect of garlic oil on typhoid bacilli is found to be twenty-four times greater than that of carbolic acid as measured by the most modern methods.

The Profile

Botanical Name	:	*Allium sativum* L.
English Names	:	Garlic, Clove Garlic.
Indian Names	:	Assamese : *Naharu*
		Bengali : *Rashun*
		Gujarati : *Lasan*
		Hindi : *Lasan*
		Kannada : *Bellulli*
		Kashmiri : *Ruhan*
		Malayalam : *Vellulli*
		Marathi : *Lusoon*
		Oriya : *Rasuna*
		Punjabi : *Lassan, Lasum*
		Sanskrit : *Lashuna*
		Tamil : *Poondu, Ullipoondu*
		Telugu : *Velluri*
		Urdu : *Lashun*

Family	:	Liliaceae.
Appearance	:	Herb of the onion family. The bulb consists of 6 to 35 bulblets called cloves enclosed in a thick, whitish, glistening and transparent jacket.
Distribution	:	All over India.
Medicinal Parts	:	Bulb.
Preparation and Dosage	:	*Juice*: 1/2 tsp of the juice pressed from the pulp, diluted with water 2 or 3 times a day. *Cold Extract*: Steep some cloves in 1/2 cup water for 6 to 8 hrs. *Powder:* 100–500 mg. *Tincture*: Soak 100 g. cloves in 250 ml. brandy for 14 days at a temperature of 85°F in a glass bottle. Strain. *Dosage*: 5 to 25 drops, several times a day as needed.

In Tradition

AILMENT

PRESCRIPTION

✤ Rheumatic disorders

: Take a garlic capsule thrice daily for a couple of months.

✤ Arteriosclerosis, hypertension, bronchial catarrh, intestinal trouble (diarrhoea, distension)

: 3 cloves of garlic, chopped and boiled in milk and taken every night.

❧ Arteriosclerosis, high blood pressure

: Tincture (see under The Profile).

❧ Blood infection, blood sugar, blood impurities, high cholesterol

: Regular intake of garlic cloves for a few days.

❧ Blood pressure

: 2 to 3 garlic cloves taken everyday.

❧ Severe digestive disorders, dysentery

: Take 3 to 6 crushed garlic cloves with honey once or twice a day.

❧ Gas, high blood pressure

: Boil 1 tsp garlic in 1 teacup milk. Take twice a day.

❧ Intestinal parasites

: 3–4 garlic cloves steeped in water or milk overnight; the liquor is drunk next day.

❧ Intestinal worms, particularly pin worms

: Cold extract (See page 18) used as an enema.

❧ Fevers due to *pitta*-aggravation

: Grind 1 tsp garlic with 20 tulsi leaves. Add 1 cup water. Boil till reduced to half. Take 2 tbsp twice daily.

❧ Earache

: Boil well 1 tsp garlic in 2 tbsp gingelly oil. Cool and filter. Use as ear drops (2 to 3 drops).

: Put 3 drops of garlic oil into the ear.

❧ Swelling in the throat : Boil some crushed garlic in water and use it for gargling.

❧ Bronchitis in children : Mix 1 tsp oil of garlic and 3 tsp honey. Let the child eat a small amount three times a day.

❧ Cold, phlegm, tropical eosinophilia : 2 garlic cloves crushed, boiled in a cup of water along with $1/2$ tsp turmeric powder.

❧ Pneumonia and tuberculosis : $1/2$ tsp garlic, boiled with 1 teacup milk and 4 teacups water, till reduced to one-fourth of the volume. This decoction is taken thrice a day.

❧ Phlegm : The filtrate as above used as a rub on chest and throat.

❧ Cold and cough : Extract 1 tsp each juice from fresh ginger, betel leaf and tulsi leaves. Add 1 tsp honey. Take 2 or 3 times a day.

❧ Cough : Grate a few garlic cloves. Mix in some honey and use 1 tsp daily.

❧ Acne, boils, corns in the foot, warts, etc. : Mash the garlic cloves and apply externally.

❧ Acne, pimples, ringworm : A couple of garlic cloves, crushed and rubbed several times a day on the affected areas. (This process is further helped by taking garlic regularly in the diet.)

❧ Infected wounds : Garlic juice with distilled water (1:3), employed as a lotion.

❧ Itch; skin-
infections : Heat 2 tbsp coconut oil and put in 1 tsp crushed garlic. Fry it till it turns red. Strain and use this oil for massaging the affected areas.

: Crush some garlic and rub it on the skin before going to bed.

❧ To avert possibility : 1/2 tsp garlic powder taken every day.
of further heart
attacks in those
who have suffered
a heart attack

Note: Individual results may vary.

A Word of Caution

Garlic, when taken in excess, heats up the body and irritates the stomach; it can cause a burning sensation during urination, and reduce spermatogenesis.

During pregnancy and lactation, excess garlic intake might cause heart-burn; it may badly affect the taste of mother's milk, which in turn, could affect the health of infants.

It is better not to eat garlic as such in the raw stage as it may 'burn' the soft tissues in the stomach; it can be eaten raw with honey or boiled in water or milk.

Garlic should never be eaten on an empty stomach, as it may cause irritation.

People with acidity problems and high *pitta* should avoid garlic.

Garlic may not be a good common usage herb for those who wish to practice yoga or meditation intensely.

The sulphur-containing volatile oil in garlic could be a skin-irritant.

In Science

Alkiewicz, J. and J. Lutomski. 1992. Study on the activity of the chloroform-extract of garlic on *Candida albicans*. *Herba Polonica* 38(2):79–84. (The efficiency of garlic against *candida* in the respiratory tracts of children.)

Amba, V. et al. 1981. Clinical evaluation of garlic capsule in chronic rheumatic disorders. *Indian J. Pharmacol.* 13:64. (Garlic capsules in a dose of one capsule thrice daily for 2 months showed significant effects on patients with different rheumatic disorders associated with pain, tenderness, swelling, range of movements, duration of morning stiffness, grip strength.)

Annapurna, Mrs. 1977. Efficiency of Lasona on rheumatic disorders. *Rheumatism* 13(1):24–27. (Garlic of comparatively greater efficacy in the treatment of rheumatic fever as compared to *Yogaraja Guggulu* and *Mahayogaraja Gugguli*.)

Augusti, K. T. and P. T. Mathew. 1973. Effect of longterm feeding of the aqueous extract of onion (*Allium cepa* L.) and garlic (*Allium sativum* L.) on normal rats. *Indian J. Exptl. Biol.* 11(3):239–241. (Water extract of garlic in a dose of 1 ml/100 g for 2 months lowered protein and lipid levels, but increased free amino acid levels of serum and liver in albino rats.)

Augusti, K. T. 1977. Hypocholesterolaemic effect of garlic (*Allium sativum* Linn). *Indian J. Expt. Biol.* 15(6):489–490. (Oral administration of water extract of garlic for hypercholesterolaemic patients for 4 months (0.5 ml per kg per day) significantly reduced cholesterol level because of sulphur-containing compound in it, which could react with SH-group systems.)

Augusti, K. T. 1996. Therapeutic value of onion (*Allium cepa* L.) and garlic (*Allium sativum* L.). *Indian J. Exp. Bio.* 34,7:634–640. (Excessive intake may interfere with haemoglobin production and may lead to lysis of RBCs.)

Bhakuni, D. S. et al. 1971. Screening of Indian plants for biological activity Pt III. *Indian J. Exptl. Biol.* 9:91–102. (Anti-inflammatory effects reported.)

Bhandari, P. R. and B. Mukerji. 1959. Garlic (*Allium sativum*) and its medicinal value. *Nagarjun* 4: 121–129. (A general account of garlic.)

Bordia, A. and H. S. Bansal. 1973. Essential oil of garlic in prevention of artherosclerosis. *Lancet* II: 1491. (Garlic juice and oil exhibit hypolipidaemic activity.)

Bordia, A. et al. 1974. Effect of the essential oil (active principle) of garlic on serum cholesterol, plasma fibrinogen, whole blood, coagulation time and fibrinolytic activity in alimentary lipaemia. *J. Assoc. Phys. India* 22:267. (Both garlic juice and oil produced significant protective action against fat-induced increased serum cholesterol.)

Chopra, R. N. et al. 1956. *Glossary of Indian Medicinal Plants.* New Delhi: Council of Scientific and Industrial Research. (Garlic's significant role in flatulence and colic.)

Dalvi, R. R. and D. K. Salunkhe. 1993. An overview of medicinal and toxic properties of garlic. *J. Mahar. Agrl. Univ.* 18(3):378–381. (A general survey on the usefulness of garlic as a medicine.)

Das, P. N. and B. N. Thakuria. 1974. Anthelmintic effect of garlic (*Allium sativum* L.) against *Ascaridia galli. Vetcol.* 14:47–52. (Worms effectively treated using garlic.)

Dixit, V. P. and S. Joshi. 1982. Effect of chronic administration of garlic (*Allium sativum*) on testicular function. *Indian J. Exptl. Biol.* 20(7):534–536. (A dose of 50 mg per rat for 45 days reduced serum cholesterol, triglyceride, phospholipid and transaminase enzyme action; it also inhibited spermatogenesis, testicular total protein and sialic acid concentration of epididymis and seminal vesicle and leydig cell function suggesting that garlic might have anti-androgenic nature of action.)

Gurdip Singh and G. N. Chaturvedi. 1974. Anticoagulant and fibrinolytic effects of garlic (*Allium sativum*) on experimental study. *J. Res. Indian Med.* (Alcoholic extract of garlic after oral administration for 7 days showed reduction in serum cholesterol.)

Hikeno, H. et al. 1986. Antihepatotonic actions of *Allium sativum* bulbs. *Planta Med.* 3, 163–168. (Allium, a volatile oil produced most remarkable hepato-protective effect against liver damage in rats.)

Jain, R. C. 1976. Onion and garlic in experimental cholesterol induced artherosclerosis. *Indian J. Med. Res.* 64(10): 1509–1515. (10 ml garlic juice extracted from 25 g garlic administered orally on artherosclerotic rabbits reduced serum lipid and cholesterol in aorta and liver.)

Jain, R. C. 1993. Anti-bacterial activity of garlic extract. *Indian J. Medical Microb.* 1(1):26–31. (Garlic as a germicidal.)

Kahloos, K. et al. 1993. Effects of garlic (*Allium sativum*) products on fungal growth and on production of some lipids *in vitro*. *Planta Med.* 59 (Suppl): 4676. (Garlic and its fungicidal properties.)

Kamanna, V. S. and Chandrasekhara. 1984. Hypocholesteremic activity of different fractions of garlic. *Indian J. Med. Res.* 79:580–583. (Garlic reduces cholesterol levels.)

Kaur, J. et al. 1981. Effect of *C. mukul, A. sativum, and A. cepa* on coaguation and fibrinolysis in experimental artherosclerosis. *Indian J. Pharmacol.* 13(1):89–90. (Garlic produced enhancement of clotting time, plasma fibrinogen clot lysis time in artherosclerotic animals.)

Maroli, S. and S. Javale. 1982. Garlic (*Allium sativum*) as a common household remedy. *Paediatr. Clin. India* 17(2):9–10. (Garlic's effect on CNS , gastro-intestinal, cardio-vascular, respiratory, locomotory and reproductive systems.)

Mirhadi, S. A. and Sudarshan Singh. 1987. Effect of garlic extract on *in vitro* uptake of $Ca2+$ and $HPO4$ $2-$ by matrix of sheep aorta.

Indian J. Exptl. Biol. 25(1):22–23. (Extract 1 ml. from 0.25 g garlic bulb completely inhibited uptake of Ca2+ and HPO4 2– when added to sheep aorta extract.)

Misra, S. B. and S. N. Dixit. 1977. Anti-fungal properties of *Allium sativum*. *Sci.& Cult.* 43(II): 487–488. (Leaf-extract *in vitro* studies against *Alternaria, Helminthosporium, Curvularia* and *Fusarium* produced complete inhibiton of fungal growth.)

Murthy, V. S. et al. 1983. Anti-microbial action and therapeutics of garlic. *J. Sci. Industr. Res.* 42(7):410–414. (Garlic as an effective bactericidal.)

Prakash, A. O. and B. Mathur. 1976. Screening of Indian plants for antifertility activity. *Indian J. Exptl. Biol.* 14(5):623–626. (Antifertility activity of garlic.)

Prasad, D. B. et al. 1966. Study of anti-inflammatory activity of some indigenous drugs in albino rats. *Indian J. Med. Res.* 54(6):582–590. ('Allisatin' administered to rats exhibited significant but low anti-inflammatory activity.)

Prasad, G. et al. 1982. Efficacy of garlic (*Allium sativum*) therapy against experimental dermatophytosis in rabbits. *Indian J. Med. Res.* 75:465-467. (Garlic showed significant curative prospect in the experimental production of the dermatophyte, *Microsporium carnis* in rabbits.)

Pushpendran, C. K. et al. 1980. Cholesterol lowering effect of *Allium* in suckling rats. *Indian J. Exptl. Biol.* 18(8):858–861. (Garlic lowers cholesterol levels.)

Raman, J. S. et al. 1978. Compounds of *lasuna* (garlic) in the prevention and treatment of cardio-vascular diseases, Report of study on human subjects. *J. Nat. Integ. Med. Ass.* 20(7):225–227. (Average blood pressure level, serum cholesterol level and blood sugar level were reduced with administration of capsule containing garlic and *swarna-bhasma* for 100 days.)

Rees, L. P. et al. 1993. Qualitative assessment of the anti-microbial activity of garlic (*Allium sativum*). *World J. Microb. & Biotech.*

9(3):303–307. (Water-extract of freeze-dried garlic inhibited the growth of bacteria, fungi and a virus.)

Sarkar, A. R. and M. K. De. 1983. Some observations on the role of garlic in the treatment of experimental hyperlipidaemia. *Calcutta Med. J.* 80(11–12):157–161. (12 weeks administration of garlic exhibited reduction in cholesterol, triglyceride and betalipoprotein of serum, suggesting that garlic is helpful in reducing hyperlipidaemia.)

Sharma, K. K. et al. 1976. Effect of raw and boiled garlic in blood cholesterol in butter fat lipaemia. *Indian J. Nutr. Dietet.* 13(1):7–10. (Reduction in cholesterol level.)

Sharma, V. D. et al. 1977. Antibacterial properties of *Allium sativum* (*in vivo* and *in vitro* studies.). *Indian J. Exptl. Biol.* 15(6)–466–468. (Water extract of garlic caused very good anti-bacterial effect against gram-negative bacteria. Marked reduction in the number of viable gram-negative bacilli per gram of rectal content was noted after oral administration of crude extract after 24 hrs of such administration and was at its minimum after repeating 4 doses of 1 ml each, once a day.)

Sreenivasamurthy, V. et al. 1962. Therapeutic usefulness of garlic. Its use in the treatment of rheumatoid arthritis. *Nat. Med. J.* 1. (Garlic in the form of syrup and an enzyme preparation in the form of powder form in capsule administered to 45 patients having rheumatic arthritis with pain and restricted movement in one or more joints. Relief reported in 32 patients.)

Weber, N. D. et al. 1992. *In vitro* virucidal effects of *Allium sativum* garlic extract and compounds. *Planta Medica* 58 (5):417–423. (Garlic's usefulness against viral diseases.)

4

Neem
Azadirachta indica

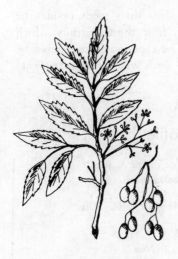

*Nimba, the great medicine
for the cure of pitta-
aggravations and for blood-
purification.*

—Priyanighantu
Haritakyadivarga

Nature's Air Purifiers

In this otherwise pollution-wrapped planet, it is heartening to note that over eighteen million neem trees, dedicated air-purifiers, are constantly engaged in releasing pure oxygen into the air, replacing toxic carbon gases.

Almost all parts of this tree can claim some or the other medicinal use. For the Hindus, it has a certain spiritual significance too. It is believed that its abundant inflorescences promote spiritual achievements.

Of Crows and Seeds

May-June is the season for neem fruits in Tamil Nadu. It is the time when a neem tree is frequented by hungry crows, which hold the fruit firmly between their claws and use their powerful beak to swallow the pulp. Eventually the skin of the fruit is dropped down as the contents are gobbled up. The entire ground below the neem tree can be seen littered with the skins. One may also find lumps of seeds deposited along with the faecal matter excreted by the crow.

Some school-children collected these 'dirty' seeds, besides the 'clean' seeds collected straightaway from the ripe fruits, which were not touched by the crow. The experiment conducted by them revealed that it is the 'dirty' seeds which germinate faster than the 'clean' ones.

The Profile

Botanical Names	:	*Azadirachta indica* A. Juss.
		Melia azaderachta L.
English Names	:	Neem, Margosa, Indian Lilac.
Indian Names	:	Bengali &
		Oriya : *Nim*
		Gujarati : *Limbro*
		Hindi : *Nim, Nimb*
		Kannada : *Bevu*
		Malayalam : *Vepa*
		Marathi : *Nimba, Limba*
		Sanskrit : *Nimba*
		Tamil : *Vembu, Veppam*
		Telugu : *Vepa*
Family	:	Meliaceae.

Appearance	:	Deciduous tree upto 12 m tall. Fissured dark grey bark. Pinnate Leaves. Flowers, small and white. Fruits, green or yellow with one seed.
Distribution	:	Almost everywhere in the plains of India and her neighbouring countries. About 20 million trees grow in South Asia.
Medicinal Parts	:	Flowers, leaves, bark, root, fruit, seed, oil.
Preparation and Dosage	:	Infusion (hot or cold), decoction, paste, powder (250–500 mg dosage), medicated ghee, medicated oil.

In Tradition

AILMENT	PRESCRIPTION
❧ Joint pains, rheumatism, ringworm, scabies, itch	: Regular massaging of body with neem oil.
❧ Biliousness, intestinal worms, phlegm	: Fry 1 tsp dried neem flowers in 1 tsp ghee and mix with 1 teacup boiled rice and eat twice or thrice a day.
❧ Piles	: Take 1 tsp of the inner bark mixed with 2 tsp jaggery powder.
❧ Excess flow of blood due to piles	: Eat 3–4 unripe neem fruits (even if it is bitter).
❧ Fever	: The leaf decoction taken with pepper powder.

❧ Dandruff, falling of hair, lice, infection in scalp

: A handful of leaves boiled in 4 teacups water. After cooling and filtering, the decoction is used for rinsing hair.

❧ Certain types of deafness

: Two drops of lukewarm neem oil put inside the ear.

❧ Earache

: Leaf juice as ear drops.

❧ Ear diseases

: The leaf decoction, when bearably warm, used as ear drops.

❧ Gum diseases, loose teeth and bad odour

: Neem twigs used as tooth brushes.

❧ Headache

: Extracted juice of leaves used as nasal drops.

❧ Headache/ stomach ache

: Neem flowers, ground and applied over head/stomach.

❧ Lice

: Grind the seeds into a fine powder and mix in some groundnut oil. Apply to the scalp. Allow it to remain overnight. Wash off next morning.

❧ Throat pain and infection

: Crush the leaves in water, remove fibre. Warm it up. Add a little honey and gargle.

❧ Swellings in the neck

: Grind finely equal quantities of tender leaf buds of neem and turmeric and apply the paste on the affected areas.

❧ Boils, glandular : Leaves ground into a paste and applied
swellings, pimples, on affected parts.
syphilitic sores,
skin eruption,
ulcers, wounds

❧ Chickenpox, : Fresh leaves ground to a paste and
smallpox and applied externally.
other skin
infections

❧ Chronic skin : Rub neem oil on affected areas.
diseases, itch,
scabies, rheu-
matism, ringworm

❧ Leprosy : Sap of the neem tree taken in daily
doses for 40 days continuously. (The
patient should also be massaged with
this sap.)

❧ Itch, skin : Grind equal quantities of neem leaves
infections, cracks and turmeric and apply on affected
in the sole areas.

❧ Lesions, open : Neem bark, boiled in water thoroughly,
wounds, etc and after cooling, used to wash the
affected parts.

❧ Skin problems : Leaves soaked in water, kept under the
sun for several hours. Regular bathing
in this infusion.

❧ Wounds : Grind into a fine paste equal quantities
of chebulic myrobalan, turmeric and
neem leaves along with a little lime
juice and apply.

31

❧ Scar due to burns   : Boil 1 teacup neem bark in 4 teacups water. Remove from fire and shake liquid. Apply the emerging froth on the affected area. Repeat several times and for several days.

Note: Individual results may vary.

A Word of Caution

Neem should be used with discretion if severe fatigue or emaciation is noticed.

Avoid excessive use of neem.

In Science

Ali, B. H. 1994. Toxicology of *Azadirachta indica. J. Ethnopharmacol.* 42(1):71–72. (Toxicological study of neem.)

Banerji, R. et al. 1977. On the triterpenes of *Azadirachta indica. Filoterapia* 48:166–169.

Bhakuni, D. S. et al. 1969. Screening of Indian plants for biological activity, Part II. *Indian J. Exptl. Biol.* 7:250. (Neem's anti-bacterial and anti-protozoal potential.)

Bhandari, P. R. and B. Mukerji. 1959. The Neem: Indian Lilac. *Pharm.* 2:21–24. (Neem's pharmaceutical uses.)

Bhattacharji, S. et al. 1953. Chemical examination of the trunk-bark of nim (*Azadirachta indica* syn. *Melia azaderachta). J. Sci. Industr. Res.* 12B:154. (The use of neem bark as medicine.)

Bose, S. 1943. *The Neem.* Hyderabad: Indian Central Seed Oil Committee. (A monograph.)

Chattopadhyay, R. R. et al. 1992. Hepato-protective activity of *Azadirachta indica* leaves on paracetamol-induced hepatic damage in rats. *Indian J. Exp. Biol.* 38(8):738–740. (Neem protects the liver.)

Chopra, R. N. et al. 1956. *Glossary of Indian Medicinal Plants.* New Delhi: Council of Scientific and Industrial Research. (Neem's use in rheumatism.)

Dixit, V. P. et al. 1992. Medicinal uses of neem (*Azadirachta indica*) in fertility regulation, diabetes and artherosclerosis. *Recent Advances Med. Aromat. and Spice Crops Today and Tomorrow.* 2:463–471. (Anti-androgenic nature of crude extracts of barks and flowers; glucose-lowering activity of neem oil; efficacy of neem oil in artherosclerosis).

Garg, G. P. et al. 1993. The gastric anti-ulcer effects of the leaves of neem tree. *Planta Med.* 59(3):215–217. (Neem as cure for ulcer.)

Garg H. S. and D. S. Bhakuni. 1984. An isoprenylated flavanone from leaves of *Azadirachta indica. Phytochemistry* 23:2115–2118. (The active principle in the leaves.)

Garg, H. S. and D. S. Bhakuni. 1984. Salannolide, a meliacin from *Azadirachta indica. Phytochemistry.* 23:2383–2385. (The active chemical principle.)

Garg, H. S. and D. S. Bhakuni. 1985. Dehydrosalannol, a tetranortriterpenoid from *Azadirachta indica* leaves. *Phytochemistry* 24:866–867. (The chemical principles behind neem's efficacy.)

Jaiswal, A. K. et al. 1994. Anxiolytic activity of *Azadirachta indica* leaf-extracts in rats. *Indian J. Exp. Biol.* 32(7):489–491.

Koul, O. et al. 1990. Properties and uses of neem, *Azadirachta indica. Can. J. Bot.* 68:1–11. (A quick survey of neem.)

Madhsudanan, K. P. et al. 1984. Negative ion mass spectra of tetranortriterpenoids isolated from Neem (*Azadirachta indica* A. Juss.). *Indian J. Chem.* 23B:1082–1087. (An acid-test.)

Mahato, S. B. et al. 1987. Constituents of *Azadirachta indica* and *Melia azaderach. Sci. & Cult.* 53(5):1–29.

Mitra, C. R. et al. 1953. Chemical examination of the root-bark of *nim* (*Azadirachta indica* syn. *Melia azaderachta*). *J. Sci. Industr. Res.* 12B:152.

Mitra, C. R. 1961. Some important characteristics of neem oil and its standardisation. *Indian Oilseed J.* 3:204–207. (A standard work.)

Moosa, J. S. 1985. A study on the crude anti-diabetic drugs used in Arabian folk-medicine. *Int. J. Crude Drug Res.* 23(3):137–145. (Neem in Arabian folk-lore.)

Murthy, K. S. et al. 1978. Preliminary study on hypoglycaemic and anti-hyperglycaemic effects of *Azadirachta indica*. *Indian J. Pharmacol* 19(3):247–250. (Water-extract of neem leaves and neem oil reduces blood sugar.)

Murthy, S. P. and M. Sirsi. 1958. Pharmacological Studies in *Melia azaderachta* Part II. Estrogenic and anti-pyretic activity of neem oil and its fractions. *Indian J. Physiol Pharmacol.* 2:456. (A study of neem oil.)

Narayanan, C. R. et al. 1969. Vepinin, a new constituent of neem oil. *Indian J. Chem.* 7:187. (A new chemical present in the oil.)

Neogi, N. G. et al. 1963. *In vitro* anthelmintic activity of some indigenous drugs. *J. Indian Med. Assoc.* 41:435. (Neem's efficacy in deworming.)

Pillai, N. R. et al. 1978. Anti-gastric ulcer activity of Nimbin. *Indian J. Med. Res.* 68:169. (Nimbin cures ulcers.)

Pillai, N. R. and G. Shanthakumari. 1981. Hypoglycaemic activity of *Melia azaderachta* Linn (Neem). *Indian J. Med. Res.* 74:931. (Neem reduces the sugar-level in diabetics.)

Pillai, N. R. and G. Shanthakumari. 1984. Effect of Nimbidin on acute and chronic gastro-duodenal ulcer models in experimental animals. *Planta Med.* 50:143. (Nimbidin shows anti-ulcer activity.)

Podder, G. and S. B. Mahato. 1985. Azadirachtanin—a new limonoid from the leaves of *Azadirachta indica*. *Heterocycles* 23:2321–2325.

Praveen, D. et al. 1993. Anti-spermatic activity of *Azadirachta indica* leaves in albino rats. *Curr. Sci.* 64(9):688–689. (Neem affects sperm production.)

Riar, S. S. et al. 1993. *Neem as a contraceptive.* Bangalore: World Neem Conference 24–28 Feb. 1993. p. 85.

Schmutterer, H. (ed.) 1995. *The Neem Tree*-Azadirachta indica *A. Juss and other Meliaceous plants.* New York: VCH Publishers Inc. (A compendium of the recent research on neem.)

Sharma, M. K. et al. 1983. Effect of neem oil on blood sugar levels of normal, hyperglycaemic and diabetic animals. *Nagarjun* 26(10):247–250. (Impact of neem oil on blood sugar.)

Shrivastava, A. K. and C. S. Chouhan. 1977. Antibacterial activity of unsaponifiable matter obtained from fixed oil of seeds of *Melia azaderach* Linn. *Indian Drug Pharmaceut. Ind.* 12(3):7. (Bacteria viz., *S. aureus, Xanth citri, Proteus spp., E. coli* and *B. subtilis* regu acted on by neem.)

Shrivastava, A. K. et al. 1981. Pharmacological studies on fruit of *Melia azaderach* Linn. *J. Res. Ayur. Sid.* II, 3:260–263. (The alkaloid obtained from the fruit can stimulate the Central Nervous System.)

Singh, N. et al. 1979. *Melia azaderachta* in some common skin disorders. *Antiseptic* 76:677. (Ringworms are eradicated in 4–8 days; a cure for eczema and scabies.)

Singh, N. et al. 1980. A clinical evaluation of anthelmintic activity of *Melia azaderachta. Antiseptic* 77(5):274. (The efficacy of neem in roundworm parasites.)

Singh, R. and R. Singh. 1972. Screening of some plant extracts for antiviral properties. *Technology* (Sindri) 9:415. (Antiviral properties of neem.)

Sinha, K. C. and S. S. Riar. 1985. Neem oil—an ideal contraceptive. *Biol. Mem.* 10 (1&2):107–114. (Neem oil prevents pregnancy.)

Subramanian, M. S. and K. K. Lakshman. 1993. *Azadirachta indica* A. Juss. stem bark as an anti-leprosy source. Bangalore: World Neem

Conference. 24–29 Feb. 1993. p. 83. (Activity of neem was found akin to that of clofzimine, dapsone and rifampicin.)

Upadhyay, S. N. et al. 1992. Immuno-modulatory effects of neem (*Azdirachta indica*) oil. *Int. J. Immunopharmacol.* 14(7):1187–1193. (Neem oil and its role.)

5

Mustard
Brassica nigra

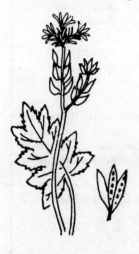

Mustard is highly useful for vitiated conditions of kapha and vata.

—Guna Paadham

The Useful Irritant

Mustard, which is an irritant, has also proved medicinally useful.

There are three distinct species of mustard: black, white and brown. All three exhibit almost the same irritant properties. It is this quality which encourages blood flow towards the surface in cases of rheumatism, sciatica, peritoritis, neuralgia and various internal inflammations.

Taken internally in small amounts—as is being done in our daily cooking (in tempering), it increases the appetite and stimulates the production of gastric juices.

The Profile

Botanical Name	:	*Brassica nigra* Koch.
English Names	:	Black Mustard, Mustard.
Indian Names	:	Bengali : *Sharsha*
		Gujarati & Hindi : *Rai, Kali Rai*
		Hindi : *Kali Sarson*
		Kannada : *Sasave*
		Kashmiri : *Aasur, Sorisa*
		Punjabi : *Banarsi Rai*
		Sanskrit : *Asuri, Bimbata*
		Tamil : *Kadugu*
		Telugu : *Avalu*
Family	:	Cruciferae.
Appearance	:	Widely cultivated annual. Leaves are alternate, lower ones bristly, upper, glabrous, lance-like, flowers are bright yellow. Black seeds develop in bulging cylindrical pods.
Distribution	:	Cultivated in Punjab, Uttar Pradesh and Tamil Nadu.
Medicinal Parts	:	Seed, oil, greens.
Other Species	:	White Mustard (*Brassica alba*); Brown Mustard (*Brassica juncea*).

In Tradition

AILMENT	PRESCRIPTION
✤ Gouty pains	: Mix mustard oil and rectified alcohol (1 part oil to 40 parts alcohol) and use as a lotion.

❧ Lumbago,
    gouty pains,
    rheumatism

: Mix mustard oil with rectified alcohol (1:40) and use as a lotion on affected parts.

❧ Stomach ache,
    stomach upset

: Mix equal quantities of mustard powder and rice flour. Add some water and boil until it reaches a paste-like consistency. Spread on a handkerchief and cover the affected parts when bearably hot.

❧ Hiccups

: Mix 2 tsp mustard powder in 1 teacup hot water. Sip.

❧ Baldness

: Boil 1 teacup mustard oil with 4 tbsp henna leaves, gradually added. Filter and bottle. Massage on the bald patches regularly.

: Grind the remains of tobacco smoked in a hookah and add to boiling mustard oil. Cool and store. Massage on the bald patches regularly.

❧ Headache,
    mental tension

: Mix equal quantities of mustard powder and rice flour. Add some water and boil until it reaches a paste-like consistency. Spread on a handkerchief and cover the affected parts when bearably hot.

❧ Migraine

: Grind $1/2$ tsp mustard seeds with 3 tsp water and strain. Instil 1 or 2 drops in nostrils.

❦ Breathing problems due to chest-congestion, cough

: Grind $1/4$ tsp seeds to a smooth paste. Mix with honey and eat.

: Mix equal quantities of mustard powder and rice flour. Add some water and boil until it reaches a paste-like consistency. Spread on a handkerchief and foment the chest and neck when bearably hot.

❦ Cough, difficulties in breathing

: Make a mustard powder-rice flour paste as above. Spread on a handkerchief and foment the chest and neck when bearably hot.

❦ Cold, flu, respiratory problems

: Take 1 teacup ground mustard in a cloth bag and boil in sufficient water. Pour the decoction into half-a-bucket hot water. Soak both feet for 20 mts.

❦ Colds, flu, respiratory problems

: Take 1 teacup ground mustard in a cloth-bag and boil in 4 teacups water. Add the decoction to a hot foot-bath.

❦ Boils, skin eruptions

: Boil 1 teacup water. Add 2 tsp ground mustard and 1 tsp sugar candy. Allow it to cool. An oil-spill-like-skin that appears on the surface is skimmed off and applied on the affected areas.

❦ Skin ailments

: Add 2 to 3 tbsp ground mustard in a bath tub of water and soak the affected parts.

| ❧ Body sluggi-
shness,
fatigue | : Add to bath water 4 teacups cold water in which 1 teacup mustard powder tied in a cloth bag had been steeped for 2–3 hrs. |

Note: Individual results may vary.

A Word of Caution

Large amounts of mustard or its prolonged use either internally or externally can cause serious irritation and inflammation.

People with sensitive skin should never let undiluted mustard oil come into contact with the skin, as it might cause blisters. Mustard can be mixed with egg-white before application.

Although packed with protein, vitamins (A, B and C), niacin, calcium, potassium, sodium and iron, mustard greens can cause serious allergy in some people.

Although mustard oil is a popular cooking medium in many parts of the country, the poisonous and mutagenic nature of isothiocyanate, a compound in mustard oil, has been the subject of controversy in recent years. Isothiocyanate is reported to have caused goitre in experimental animals.

In Science

Ahmad, P. and A. J. Muztav. 1971. Effect of allyl-thiocyanate on the thyroid glands of rat. *Pakistan J. Biochem.* 5:72–77; *Chem. Abstr.* 77:160858. (Isothiocyanate in mustard oil which is considered poisonous and mutagenic induces goitre in laboratory animals.)

Eckey, E. W. 1954. *Vegetable Fats and Oils.* New York: Reinhold Publishing Corporation.

Frawley, D. and V. Lad. 1994. *The Yoga of Herbs.* Delhi. (Mustard's medicinal importance.)

HOME REMEDIES

Lust, John. 1974. *The Herb Book*. New York: Bantam Books. (Mustard as a home remedy.)

Pruthi, J. S. 1976. *Spices and Condiments*. New Delhi. p. 160–164. (Notes on mustard.)

Rajendra Prasad, Y. et al. 1993. Anti-microbial studies on the seed oil of *Brassica juncea*. *Filoterapia* 64(4):373–374. (Both gram-positive and gram-negative bacteria are acted on by mustard oil.)

Swern, D. 1979. *Bailey's Industrial Oils and Fat Products*. Revised edn. New York: John Wiley & Sons. (Mustard oil in industry.)

Tandon, G. L. & G. Lal. 1960. Chemical Composition of Mustard (Mustard Flour or Ground Mustard) and Mustard Compounds. *Indian Food Packer 14* (8):15–18. (The chemistry of irritability.)

Tandon G. L. et at. 1961. Quality of Indian Black Mustard. *Indian Food Packer* 15 (1):11–14. (The chemical personality.)

Tandon, G. L. & G. S. Siddappa. 1963. Mustard (Mustard flour) and Mustard Compounds. *Indian Oilseeds Journal* (1):55–59. (Chemical analysis of pungent factors.)

6

Chilli

Capsicum frutescens

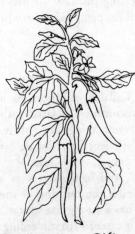

Chillies are the answer to vitiated conditions of kapha and vata.

—Svayamkriti

Portuguese Gift

What imparts the so-called 'Indianness' to the cuisine of the subcontinent is that green, slender fruit called chilli.

Some four hundred years ago Indians were not familiar with chillies at all—the fruit 'which looked like the tail of a scorpion and tasted like its sting.'

It was the Portuguese who brought chillies along with their cannons to India.

Fruit of the Sun

Chilli is metaphorically referred to in Sanskrit as *Marichi-Palam*, the Sun's Fruit. Like black pepper (*marich*), chilli is also believed to be as hot as the sun.

The Varieties

There are two important species: white-flowered *Capsicum annuum* and the greenish-white (and more pungent) *Capsicum frutescens.*

There are several varieties of chilli, varying in shape, size, colour and pungency factors. The level of pungency of a species depends upon the concentration of capsaicin in the fruit.

A variety, popular in Tamil Nadu, called *Oosi Milagai* (the Pin Chilli), true to its name, has a piercing bite. At the other extreme, you have the most harmless bell pepper, *Simla Mirch* or *Kudai Milagai* (the Umbrella Chilli).

Chillies in Cuisine

The pungency factor of the chillies stimulates salivation. As a result, the starchy staple food of the subcontinent is laced with the enzyme amylase, which ensures proper breaking down of the complex carbohydrates. This may be the scientific rationale for its inclusion in the diet. There are, of course, other reasons.

Chilli is rich in Vitamins A and C, and hence serves as a good vitamin supplement too. It facilitates the burning of the toxins accumulated in the colon. As it has a strong haemostatic action, it could be used profitably in acute cases to arrest bleeding.

It is reported that the Cancer Research Institute, Adyar, Chennai, has discovered that green chilli retards cancer.

Some researchers 'credit' the fecundity of the third world to chillies.

The Profile

Botanical Names	: *Capsicum frutescens* L. *Capsicum annuum* L.
English Names	: Africa Pepper, American Pepper, Zanzibar Pepper, Spanish Pepper, Capsicum, Chili Pepper, Red Pepper, Cockspur Pepper, Goat's Pepper, Pod Pepper, Bird Pepper.

Indian Names	:	Bengali & Oriya	: *Lanka*
		Gujarati	: *Marcha*
		Hindi & Urdu	: *Lal Mirch*
		Kannada	: *Menssina Kayi*
		Kashmiri	: *Martsu, Waungam*
		Malayalam	: *Mulaku*
		Marathi	: *Mirchi*
		Tamil	: *Milagai*
		Telugu	: *Mirapakayi*

Origin : Native of the West Indies and tropical America.

Appearance : The plant grows to a height of 3 feet. Stem is glabrous and woody near the base and branched near the top. Leaves are lance-like. Flowers are white to yellow and drooping. The ripe fruit is a many-seeded pod with a leathery outside in various shades of red or yellow.

Distribution : Cultivated all over India in about 9 lakh hectares.

Medicinal Parts : Fruit (fresh or dried).

Preparation and Dosage : *Infusion:* $1/2$ to 1 tsp red pepper per cup of boiling water. Dosage: 1 tsp at a time, warm. Powder: For acute conditions, take 3 to 10 grains; for chronic conditions: 1 to 3 grains.

In Tradition

AILMENT | PRESCRIPTION

❧ Abdominal pain : Make a chutney of 2 tsp coriander seeds, 1 tsp ginger, 1 green chilli and 2 tbsp grated coconut. Eat with steamed rice.

❧ Nausea, diarrhoea : Make a paste of 1 green chilli along with 2 tbsp lime juice and $1/2$ tsp camphor. Take $1/4$ tsp of this paste. (Advisable only in an emergency.) (*Note:* There will be a burning sensation.)

❧ Throat irritation : Boil 10 roses in 1 teacup water. Add to the filtrate 3 pinches of red chilli powder. Gargle a few times when bearably warm. (*Note:* There will be a burning sensation.)

❧ Swellings in the neck region : Make a paste of a few green chillies by grinding them in water. Apply this paste on the exterior of the throat before going to bed. (*Note:* There will be a burning sensation.)

Note: Individual results may vary.

A Word of Caution

The chilli's sting is well-known. Its quality is *rajasic.* It may cause mental disturbances when taken in excess. Those who desire mental peace should therefore keep the chilli away. The ingenious Indian cuisine however beautifully neutralizes the adverse effects of chilli by adding coolants like coriander leaves and powder, coconut milk, khuskhus seeds, etc.

Those who suffer from ulcers, gastritis, enteritis, and other inflammatory conditions should avoid chilli.

Long-term use of red chilli can promote haemorrhaging.

While on the one hand chilli could be of help in cases of heart weaknesses or heart attack (for revival), it can also aggravate *pitta* conditions leading to heart attack.

Excessive consumption of chilli may cause gastro-enteritis and kidney damage. Prolonged application to the skin can cause dermatitis and raise blisters.

In Science

Awasthi, D. N. and B. P. Singh. 1973. Isolation and identification of capsaicin and allied compounds in chilli. *Proc. Indian Acad. Sci.* 77B(5):196–201. (Research on capsaicin.)

Awasthi, D. N. et al. 1976. Ascorbic acid content and its correlation with the age and size of developing fruits of some chilli varieties. *Progve. Hort.* 7(4):15–18. (On the significant Vitamin C content.)

Bajaj, K. L. et al. 1977. Seasonal variations in ascorbic acid, dry matter and phenolic content of chillies as affected by fruit maturity. *Veget. Sci.* 4(2):129–133.

Bajaj, K. L. et al. 1978. Varietal variation in the capsaicin content in *Capsicum annuum* fruits. *Veget. Sci.* 5(1):23–29. (On varietal differences in bio-synthesis of capsaicin.)

Biswas, H. G. and K. L. Das. 1939. *Ind Jour. Med. Res. 27.* (Vitamin C content of chillies, onion and garlic both raw and when boiled in water.)

Clarke, I. M. C. 1993. Peppering Pain. *Lancet* 342 (8880):1130. (Topical application of capsaicin is worth a try especially when the pain is typical of differentiation and there is a clear organic aetiology.)

Farnsworth, N. R .and A. B. Segelman. 1971. Hypoglycaemic plants. *Tile and Till* 57(3):52–56. (Hypoglycaemic properties reported.)

Gal, I. E. 1972. Extraction of antibiotic capsicidin from mature *Capsicum annuum* seeds by a simple method. *Z. Lebensm.-Unters.-Forsch.* 148:286–289; *Chem. Abstr.* 77:92319. (In German.)

Kaur, G. et al. 1980. Studies on variations in protein and mineral contents in dried red fruits of chilli varieties. *Indian Fd. Pack.* 24(1):21–23. (An analysis.)

Lille, J. and E. Ramerez. 1935. *Chem. Abstr.* 4836. (Pharmacodynamic action of chillies.)

Lust, J. 1974. *The Herb Book.* New York: Bantam Books. (Chilli as a remedy.)

Maga, J. A. 1975. Capsicum. *CRC Crit. Rev. Food Sci. Nutr.* 6:177–179. (High levels of consumption of chillies induce stomach ulcers and cirrhosis of liver in experimental animals.)

Ramanujan, S. and D. K. Tirumalachar. 1966. Component analysis of capsaicin content in chillies. *Indian J. Gen. Pl. Br.* 26(2):227–229. (A chemical report.)

Rampal, S. 1978. A note on vitamin C content in chillies. *Indian J. Hort.* 35(4):373–374. (Chillies are a rich source of Vitamin C.)

Sethi, S. C and J. S. Agarwal. 1952. Stabilization of Edible Fats by Spices and Condiments—Part I. *J. Sci. Industr. Res.* 11B:46. (Red chillies effectively check the development of rancidity in vegetable oils.)

Solanke, T. F. 1973. The effect of red pepper—*Capsicum frutescens*—on gastric acid secretion. *J. Surg. Res.* 15:385–390. (Consumption of red pepper may aggravate the symptoms of duodenal ulcer.)

Windholz, M. ed. 1976. *The Merck Index—An Encyclopaedia of Chemicals and Drugs.* NJ. Rahway: Merck & Co. Inc. (Body-temperature, flow of saliva and gastric juices stimulated by chillies.)

7

Papaya

Carica papaya

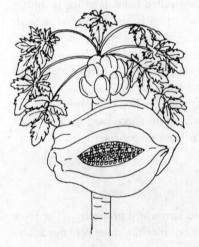

Papaya cures haemorrhagic diseases, and is especially beneficial in the treatment of piles.

—Dravyaguna

Nearly every inch of a papaya tree possesses medicinal properties.

Papaya Leaves

The leaves contain carpaine, an alkaloid which is reported to show anti-tumour activity *in vitro* against leukaemia. Traditionally, the leaves are used in relieving muscle pain and curing festering wounds, ringworm, etc.

Papaya Root

The root is abortifacient and diuretic. Internally, it is administered for checking irregular bleeding from the uterus.

The Papaya Fruit

The papaya fruit is loaded with carotenes (which take part in the production of Vitamin A inside the human body), potassium, (which helps in the maintenance of balance between fluids inside and outside human cells) and enzymes (which work as catalysts in innumerable chemical reactions constantly taking place inside the human body).

It contains a powerful enzyme called papain, which is similar to pepsin found in our stomach. It prevents improper protein breakdown in the system, thus preventing many allergies and stomach ailments.

The unripe fruit is laxative and diuretic. The dried and salted fruit reduces enlarged liver and spleen.

The ripe fruit is useful in cases of bleeding piles and dyspepsia. It helps in removing urinary concretions and is used for treatment of haemoptysis and wounds in the urinary tract.

The Papaya Seeds

The seeds possess antibiotic and antifungal properties. The juice of seeds is administered in cases of bleeding piles, enlarged liver and spleen conditions.

Like the legendary apple, a papaya a day can also keep the doctor away.

The Profile

Botanical Name	:	*Carica papaya* L.
English Names	:	Pawpaw, Custard Apple, Melon Tree, Papaya.
Indian Names	:	Hindi : *Papita* Tamil : *Pappali*

Other Vernacular Names	: *Penpe, Parisha, Arand, Kharbuza.*
Family	: Caricaceae.
Appearance	: A tree having soft wood with palm-like leaves. Male and female flowers are on separate trees. The fruit is a large, oblong or nearly spherical fleshy berry with yellow-orange rind like a gourd.
Distribution	: Cultivated chiefly in Uttar Pradesh, Punjab, Rajasthan, Gujarat, Maharashtra and Tamil Nadu.
Medicinal Parts	: Leaves, fruits (ripe or unripe), latex.

In Tradition

AILMENT	PRESCRIPTION
❧ Muscle pain	: Warm the leaf over the fire and apply on affected parts.
❧ Anaemia constipation, eye-diseases, intestinal worms	: Eat papayas frequently.
❧ Enlargement of the spleen	: Skin the ripe papaya fruit, cut into pieces and immerse in vinegar for a week. Take about 2 tbsp of this preserved fruit twice daily.
❧ Liver and spleen inflamma- tion	: Take every day a big slice of papaya with 1 tsp of honey. (Avoid sugar, starch, fat, meat and constipative foods.)

❧ Jaundice : A fine paste of tender leaves ($1/2$ tsp) is taken with some water.

❧ Urinary com-
plaints : An infusion of tender leaves is taken once or twice a day.

❧ To increase milk
flow in lactating
mothers : Eat cooked unripe fruits frequently.

❧ Dead, flaky skin
on face, freckles : Take a ripe papaya slice and mash the pulp. Use it as a face pack overnight.

❧ Freckles : Apply fresh milky juice of papaya on affected parts and allow it to dry for at least half an hour.

❧ Festering wounds : Apply a little castor oil on a portion of leaf. Warm it slightly over a flame. When bearably warm, dress the wounds with it.

❧ Dressing for foul
wounds : Fresh leaves are applied as a poultice for sores.

❧ Ringworm : Express fresh papaya leaf juice and apply frequently on the affected areas.

Note: Individual results may vary.

Plant's Name: Is It All Greek and Latin?

As the local name of any plant may cause confusion in identification, internationally each plant is known only by a Latin or Latinized name.

The binomial system uses a pair of such names. In the case of papaya which has the Latin name *Carica papaya*, the first of the two words represents the generic (genus) name and the second the specific (species) name. An abbreviation of the author's name is also added to this as a convention. Thus 'L' in *Carica papaya* L. indicates the name of the Swedish botanist, Linnaeus, who is the author.

A Formula for Home-Made Conditioner!

If you beat the papaya leaf in a bucketful of water, you will get rich lather, thanks to its saponin content. You can use this water along with the lather for washing your hair. This is a very effective and inexpensive home-made conditioner.

In Science

Agharkar, S. P. 1953. *Medicinal Plants - Gazeteer of Bombay State.* (Revised Series) Volume: General—A. Botany. Bombay. Part I, p. 54. (Papaya's significant nutritional value.)

Bose, T. K. ed. 1985. *Fruits of India, Tropical and Sub-Tropical.* Calcutta: Naya Prokash. (The importance of inclusion of papaya in the diet.)

Burkil, I. H. 1935. *A Dictionary of the Economic Products of the Malay Peninsula.* 2 vols. London. (The papaya in Malaysia.)

Dastur, J. F. *Medicinal Plants of India and Pakistan.* Bombay: D. B. Tarporevala & Sons.

Evans, D. A. and R. K. Raj. 1988. Extract of Indian plants as mosquito larvicides. *Indian J. Med. Res.* 88:38. (Larvicides from the papaya plant.)

Henry, T. A. 1949. *The Plant Alkaloids.* 4th edn. London: J & A Churchill Ltd.

Irvine, 1961. *Woody Plants of Ghana with Special Reference to their Uses.* London: Oxford University Press.

Kirtikar, K. R. and B. D. Basu. 1935. *Indian Medicinal Plants.* Revised by E. Blatter et al. 2nd edn. 4 vols. Allahabad II: 1098.

Lohia, N. K. et al. 1993. Induction of reversible antifertility with a crude ethanol extract of *Carica papaya* seeds in albino male rats. *Int. J. Pharmacognosy* 30(4):308–320. (Papaya seeds as abortifacient.)

Osato, J. A. et al. 1992. Anti-microbial and anti-oxidant activities of unripe papaya. *Life Sci.* 53(17):383–9. (The bactericidal properties of unripe fruit.)

Quisumbing, E. 1951. Medicinal Plants of Philippines. *Technical Bulletin* No. 16.

Rama Rao, M. 1914. *Flowering Plants of Travancore, Trivandrum.* Dehra Dun: International Book Distributors.

8

Cinnamon

Cinnamomum zeylanicum

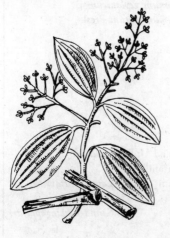

Cinnamon fights toxins.

—Abhidaana Manjari

A Spice from Sri Lanka

The botanical name *zeylanicum* of this plant refers to its original birthplace, Sri Lanka.

However, historical and archaeological findings testify that cinnamon had reached the royal treasuries of faraway Egypt by as early as the fifth century B.C. This confirms the amazing tie-ups that existed through the age-old sea routes between the two continents.

Cinnamon as a Medicine

The stem-bark which is used as a flavouring agent also possesses medicinal properties. Oil obtained from this is used as a carminative, antiseptic and as an astringent.

Cinnamon along with cardamom and bay leaf form the Three Great Aromatics, which help in digestion and absorption. Cinnamon strengthens the heart, stimulates the kidneys and harmonizes the flow of circulation.

The Profile

Botanical Names	:	*Cinnamomum zeylanicum* B.
		Cinnamomum verum Presl.
English Name	:	Cinnamon.
Indian Names	:	Bengali,
		Gujarati,
		Hindi,
		Marathi,
		Oriya,
		Punjabi and Urdu : *Dalchini*
		Kannada and
		Malayalam : *Lavangpattai*
		Sanskrit : *Darushila*
		Tamil : *Sanna-Lavangapattai*
Family	:	Lauraceae.
Appearance	:	Evergreen tree with large leathery leaves and minute flowers in hairy clusters.
Distribution	:	Nilgiris, South Kanara, Malabar, Assam and Kumaon.
Medicinal Parts	:	The bark of the stem and the oil obtained from it are useful as antiseptics, astringents and carminatives; the oil obtained from the leaves is used as a flavouring agent and for local application on certain rheumatic pains.

In Tradition

AILMENT	PRESCRIPTION

Anaemia : Dissolve ground cinnamon (1 tsp) and 2 tsp honey in 2 cups pomegranate juice. *Dosage:* $1/2$ cup.

Nausea : Eat a pinch of cinnamon powder.

Diarrhoea : Combine 1 tsp each powdered ginger, cumin and cinnamon with honey and make into a thick paste. Take 1 tsp thrice daily.

Bad breath : Boil 1 tsp cinnamon in 1 teacup water. Cool. Use frequently as a mouth wash.

: Make an infusion of cinnamon, cardamom and bay leaves (equal parts) and take 1 tsp in a cup of water twice or thrice a day. In addition, cleanse the mouth with liquorice powder and chew some saunf.

Bed breath or halitosis : Chew a piece of cinnamon bark folded in a betel leaf.

Loss of taste sensitivity in the tongue : Rub on the tongue a mixture of finely powdered cinnamon and honey and allow it to remain for sometime.

Headache : Make a fine powder of 1 tsp each saffron, gum myrrh and cinnamon. Add water and make a paste. Put this paste onto a clean piece of cotton cloth and apply to one or both temples.

❧ Headache, caused by exposure to cold air : Mix 1 tsp finely ground cinnamon in 1 tsp water and apply on the affected parts.

❧ To increase lactation (it indirectly helps delay menstruation) : $1/2$ tsp finely ground cinnamon taken every night along with 1 teacup milk.

❧ To delay menstruation after childbirth : Take a small piece of cinnamon in powdered form every night along with milk, after delivery. (*Note:* This treatment is reported to delay menstruation by 15 to 20 months, besides helping secretion of breast milk. Prolonged breastfeeding is reported to check the restarting of menstruation.)

❧ Blockage in nose due to cold and phlegm : Sniff a mixture of finely powdered cinnamon, black pepper, cardamom and black cumin seeds, all in equal parts, frequently.

❧ Cough : Prepare a tea of $1/2$ tsp ginger, with $1/4$ tsp each cinnamon and cloves per cup of water. Sweeten with 1 tsp honey and drink.

❧ Common cold, influenza, sore throat : Boil $1/2$ tsp each finely powdered cinnamon and black powdered pepper in 1 teacup water. Add honey and drink.

❧ Acne, blackheads, pimples : Mix 1 tsp lime juice in 1 tsp finely ground cinnamon powder and apply on affected areas frequently.

❧ To improve   : Add a pinch of cinnamon powder
  the complexion   to $1/2$ tsp honey and apply on the face
                        every night.

❧ To improve com-   : Take a mixture of 1 tsp honey and a
  plexion; to im-   pinch of finely powdered cinnamon
  prove memory;   every night regularly.
  this treatment
  strengthens
  nerves

❧ Cold, cancer of   : Boil $1/2$ tsp cinnamon bark, broken
  stomach, rectum   into bits in $11/2$ cups water for 10 mts.
  and uterus   Strain and sweeten with honey and take
                        twice daily.

❧ Sleeplessness   : Boil $1/2$ tsp cinnamon in 1 teacup water
                        for 5 mts, strain and sweeten with
                        honey. Take twice daily.

Note: Individual results may vary.

In Science

Arctander, S. 1960. *Perfume and Flavour Materials of Natural Origin.*
    New Jersey: Elizabeth.

Atal, C. K. and B. M. Kapur ed. 1977. *Cultivation and Utilization of
    Medicinal and Aromatic Plants.* Jammu-Tawi: Regional Research
    Laboratory, Council of Scientific and Industrial Research.
    (Horticultural and economic uses of cinnamon.)

Chopra, R. N. et al. 1958. *Indigenous Drugs of India.* 2nd edition.
    U. N. Calcutta: Dhar & Sons. p. 126. (Cinnamon and its medicinal
    value.)

Dastur, J. F. 1950. *Medicinal Plants of India and Pakistan.* Bombay: Taraporevala. p. 81. (Medicinal properties of cinnamon.)

Guenther, E. 1948–1952. *The Essential Oils.* 6 vols. New York: D. van Nostrand Co. Inc. (Cinnamon oil, its chemical composition and commercial uses.)

Kirtikar, K. R. and B. D. Basu. 1935. *Indian Medicinal Plants.* Revised by E. Blatter et al. 2nd edition. vol.III. Allahabad. p 2149. (Cinnamon as a medicinal plant.)

Purseglove, J. W. et al. 1981. *Spices.* Tropical Agriculture Series. 2 vols. New York: Longman Inc.

Sethi, S. C. and J. S. Agarwal. 1952. Stabilization of Edible Fats by Spices and Condiments. Part I. *J. Sci. Industr. Res* 11B:46. (Cinnamon leaf effectively checks rancidity in vegetable oils.)

Watt, J. M. and M. G. Breyer-Brandwijk. 1962. *The Medicinal and Poisonous Plants of Southern and Eastern Africa.* 2nd edition. Edinburgh. p. 531. (Curative properties of cinnamon.)

Lime

Citrus aurantiifolia

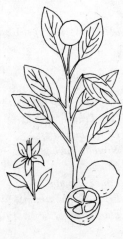

*Lime adds beauty and
prosperity to a house.*

—Matsya Purana
255, 24. (8th Century A.D.)

The Medicinal Role of Taste

Lime is an easily available fruit, sour in taste. The sour taste
which is due to the presence of various acids is believed to be the
reason for its medicinal value.

Sour taste, in terms of herbalism, acts as a stimulant, promotes
digestion, increases appetite and is a carminative (helps dispel
flatus). It nourishes all tissues, except reproductive tissues (*shukla
dhatu*).

Very much like amla, this fruit is also the poor person's rich
source of Vitamin C.

In Siddha literature, wherever an unspecified fruit (*kani*) is called for, the practitioner uses lime fruit in preference to all others.

The Profile

Botanical Names	:	*Citrus aurantiifolia* (Christm) Swing. *Limonia aurantiifolia* Christm. *Limonia acidisima* Houtt. *C. Lima* Lun. *C. acida* Roxb. *C. medica* var. *acida* Hook. f. *C. hystrix* subsp. *acida* Engl.	
English Names	:	Lime, Acid Lime, Sour Lime.	
Indian Names	:	Bengali	: *Kaghzi Lebu, Lebu, Pati Lebu*
		Gujarati	: *Khata Limbu*
		Hindi & Urdu	: *Nimbu, Kaghzi Nimbu*
		Kannada	: *Limbe, Nimbe*
		Malayalam	: *Erumich Naratham*
		Tamil	: *Elumitchai*
Family	:	Rutaceae.	
Appearance	:	A shrub or small tree.	
Distribution	:	Cultivated nearly all over India, particularly in Andhra Pradesh, Maharashtra, Karnataka, Assam, Bihar, Uttar Pradesh, Punjab, West Bengal, Madhya Pradesh and Rajasthan.	
Medicinal Parts	:	Fruits, leaves, roots.	
Preparation	:	Juice, dried rind.	

In Tradition

AILMENT	PRESCRIPTION
✹ Whitlow	: Make a hole in the lime and insert the affected finger and use it as a bandage.
✹ Pain in knee joint, bone joint, etc	: Cut the lemons into small pieces. Tie them in a cotton cloth. Dip this in hot gingelly oil, and foment the affected joints when bearably hot.
✹ Sprain, swelling	: Grind lime leaves into a fine paste. Mix it with an equal quantity of butter. Apply on the affected areas.
✹ Swelling and pain in legs, hand, ankle, etc	: Mix equal quantities of castor oil and lime juice. Massage the affected area with this mixture. (Also drink 1 cup warm water mixed with lime juice and honey.)
✹ Diabetes	: Mix 2 tsp lime juice in 4 tsp amla juice and 1 tsp honey. Take in the morning on an empty stomach.
✹ High blood pressure	: Mix 1 tsp lime juice in 1 teacup butter-milk. Drink frequently.
✹ Colic, diarrhoea, dysentery	: Pour over a handful of roots 1 teacup hot water and drink the infusion.
✹ Dysentery	: Mix 2 tsp lime juice and 2 tsp sugar with 1 cup of water and drink.

❧ Jaundice,
sore throat

: Pour over a handful of leaves 1 teacup hot water and take the infusion.

❧ Haemorrhoids

: Juice of 1 lime fruit mixed with 1 teacup water, used as a retention enema.

❧ *Pitta*-aggravation,
to promote regularity and prevent constipation

: Take lime juice in a glass of warm water at daybreak.

❧ Feverishness,
nausea, etc

: Mix 1 teacup fresh lemon juice in tender coconut water and drink.

❧ Baldness,
not due to
hereditary factors

: Mix 2 teacups salt and 4 tbsp pepper powder in $1/2$ teacup lime juice. Leave it under the sun for 3 days to dry out thoroughly. Once dry, powder and bottle. *Dose:* 1 tsp mixed in water, applied on bald patches at bedtime. Wash off the next morning. (*Note:* Avoid using any soap or shampoo.)

❧ Bad breath,
ulcer in mouth

: Drink lime juice in warm water after frequent gargling. Repeat.

❧ Bleeding from
the nose due to
body heat

: Lemon juice dropped into nostrils.

❧ Blond hair
(To give blond
highlights)

: Mix the strained juice of 2 limes in an equal amount of warm water and rinse hair with it. Leave on for 15 mts and sit in the sun if possible. Then rinse out.

❧ Earache

: Mix a few drops of lime juice in 1 tsp lukewarm water. Put 4 drops of this into the ear.

❧ Early stages of cataract

: Mix 1 tsp rose water with 1 tsp fresh lime juice. Add 10 drops of this to the eyes.

❧ Eye diseases

: One drop of lime juice put into the eyes every morning.

❧ Gum bleeds

: Drink often lime juice in water. Simultaneously massage the gum frequently with coconut oil.

❧ Hair loss, premature greying of hair

: Mix dried rind of lime, with shikakai, curry leaves, seeds of fenugreek and green gram—all in equal quantities. Powder it and use for washing hair.

: Grind 1 tbsp each pulp of amla with lime juice. Massage this into the hair before going to bed. Wash it next morning.

❧ Headache, stomach ache

: Take 1/2 tsp powdered leaves along with 1 tsp honey.

❧ Toothache

: Pound some asafoetida in a mortar and pestle and add some lime juice. Heat it slightly. Soak a piece of cotton and hold it on the affected area.

❧ Watering in the eyes

: Just touch the eye lids with a lime fruit softly several times.

❧ Yellow discolouration of teeth

: Mix salt with finely powdered rind of lime. Use this as toothpowder frequently.

🌿 Throat pain   : Mix 1 tbsp each lime juice **and honey** and swallow tiny amounts slowly.

🌿 Epilepsy, nervous-   : Apply fresh lime juice on the head.
   ness, mental   Massage well before showering off.
   diseases

🌿 To facilitate the   : Mix 3 tsp lime juice with 1/4 tsp
   delivery of babies   powdered black pepper and 1 tsp honey along with 1 cup water and drink for 3 months.

🌿 Common cold   : Squeeze one fruit in a glass of hot water and add 1 tsp honey and 2 tbsp brandy. Drink before retiring to bed.

🌿 Whooping cough   : Mix equal quantities of the juices of lime, ginger and onion. Take 2 tbsp thrice a day.

🌿 Black dots,   : Apply fresh lime juice on the affected
   blemishes,   areas before going to bed. Wash them
   pimples   with warm water next morning.

🌿 Cracks in the sole,   : Finely grind a handful of henna leaves
   burning sensation   and add 2 tbsp lime juice. Stir and
   in the feet   apply on the feet.

🌿 Burns and scalds   : Combine 4 tsp each lime juice and coconut oil and rub until the mixture turns white. Apply on affected parts.

☙ Itching and burn-
ing sensations in
the skin, psoriasis,
skin-infections, etc

: Lime juice, diluted in water and used
as soap.

☙ Discoloured skin,
freckles

: Apply lime juice or cut lime peel
directly to the skin. Wash off after
15 mts. (If the skin is dry, use a skin-
conditioner afterwards.)

☙ Lice

: Mix 1 tsp lime juice with 1 tsp garlic
paste and apply on head.

☙ Marks left by
pimples on the
face

: Mix equal quantities of lime juice,
sandalwood powder and coconut oil
and apply on the face before retiring
to bed.

☙ Pimples

: Dry the young tender leaves of the lime
tree. Powder finely and mix with
turmeric powder (1:1). Use it as soap
to clean the face.

☙ Prevention of
skin infections

: Slice a lime fruit and rub the juice
all over the body before showering.

☙ Skin diseases

: Grind 1 tbsp each turmeric and
mustard seeds into a fine paste. Mix
1 tsp lime juice. Apply on affected parts.

☙ Wounds

: Grind into a fine paste equal quantities
of chebulic myrobalan, turmeric and
neem leaves along with some lime juice
and apply on wounds.

☙ Dehydration

: Add 1/4 tsp salt, 3 tsp brown sugar
and 2 tsp lime juice to 1 teacup of
water, mix well and drink.

| | : Add 2 tsp lime juice to 1 teacup water containing 1/4 tsp salt and 3 tsp cane sugar (brown sugar). Mix and drink. |

🌢 Dizziness, stomach distress : Take 1 tsp lime juice in hot water.

🌢 Indigestion, giddiness, nausea, etc : Soak cumin seeds in lime juice overnight. Keep this mixture under the sun till completely dry. Bottle it. Chew 1/2 tsp of this mixture and drink a glass of warm water.

🌢 Enlargement of spleen, giddiness, jaundice, nausea, piles, vomiting due to indigestion, etc : Frequent intake of lime juice.

🌢 Obesity : Mix lime juice with honey and water. Drink a glass of this every morning. Mix 3 tsp lime juice with 1/4 tsp powdered black pepper and 1 tsp honey along with 1 cup water and drink for 3 months.

: Take 1 tsp lime juice with 1 teacup water in the morning on an empty stomach.

: Mix 1/2 tsp black pepper powder in 1 tsp honey and 3 tsp lime juice. Add 1 cup water and drink daily.

🌢 To prevent mosquito bite : Apply lime juice diluted with water on body.

Note: Individual results may vary.

A Word of Caution

Prolonged and excessive use of lime is reported to affect normal reproductive functions.

In Science

Aiyappa, K. M. and K. C. Srivastava. 1965. *Oranges, Lemons and Limes*. New Delhi: Krishi Bhavan. (The *Citrus* Family and its economic importance.)

Bhag Singh. 1981. *Establishment of the First Gene Sanctuary in India for Citrus in Garo Hills*. New Delhi: Concept Publishing Co.

Bhattacharya, S. C. and S. Dutta. 1956. *Classification of Citrus fruits in Assam*. New Delhi: ICAR. Scientific Monograph No. 20. (*Citrus* varieties.)

Deshmukh, P. P. ed. 1984. *State-level Summer Institute in Fruit Nursery Practices: A Compilation of Lectures*. Akola: University Dept. of Horticulture. Punjabrao Krishi Vidya Peeth.

Duke, J. A. 1986. *Isthmian Ethno-Botanical Dictionary*. 3rd edition. Jodhpur: Scientific Publisher. p. 55.

Gopalan, C. et al. 1971. *Nutritive value of Indian Foods*. National Institute of Nutrition. Reprinted 1972. Hyderabad: ICMR. p. 85. (The nutritive value of lime.)

Quisumbing, E. 1951. Medicinal Plants of the Philippines. *Technical Bulletin* 16:449.

Randhawa, G. S. and K. C. Srivastava. 1986. *Citriculture in India*. Delhi: Hindustan Publishing Corporation.

Tanaka, T. ed. 1976. *Tanaka's Cyclopaedia of Edible Plants of the World*. ed. S. Nakro. Tokyo: Keigaku Publishing Co. (Lime: properties and uses.)

10

Coconut
Cocos nucifera

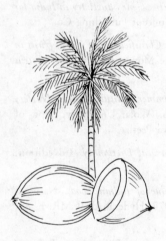

Coconut adds beauty and prosperity to a house.

—Matsya Purana
255, 24. (8th Century A.D.)

The Ideal Food

Coconut is considered to be the ideal food for human beings. The reason: the arrival of *Homo sapiens* on the planet is reported to coincide with the appearance of coconut palms.

In traditional households, coconut is strongly recommended for the expectant mother as it provides all the essential ingredients such as vitamins, minerals and enzymes for the growing foetus. Coconut is considered a great preventive medicine. It prevents the occurrence of smallpox, intestinal infections, tumours, etc.

The Oil

There are two ways of extracting oil from the plant.

Commercially, oil is extracted by crushing copra, the kernel of the dried coconut fruit. For medicinal use and also for use as hair oil, oil obtained by boiling coconut is, however, recommended by the native physicians.

The Profile

Botanical Name	:	*Cocos nucifera* L.
English Name	:	Coconut.
Indian Names	:	Hindi : *Nariyal* Tamil : *Thengai*
Family	:	Palmaceae.
Appearance	:	A common, tall palm.
Distribution	:	Cultivated chiefly in peninsular India, in Kerala, Tamil Nadu and Karnataka.
Medicinal Parts	:	Leaf, fruit, oil.

In Tradition

AILMENT	PRESCRIPTION
❧ Pain in hips	: Extract some coconut milk and cook fenugreek leaves in it. Add the contents of an egg to it and eat 2 or 3 times a day.
❧ Stomach ulcer	: Drink frequently tender coconut water and milk extracted from the kernel.

✤ Contusions : Mix 1 tbsp old grated coconut with some turmeric powder (1:1) and put it in a small cloth bag (or in a cotton pouch). Now, warm the bag over a hot plate and use it for fomenting the contusions.

✤ Hair loss : Mix 1 tbsp white powder of sweet flag in $1/2$ teacup cold coconut milk. Massage into the scalp frequently.

✤ Hair loss, skin-irritations : Massage with coconut oil everyday.

✤ Mouth ulcer : Mix some coconut milk with honey and massage the gums 3 to 4 times a day.

: Gargle with (or apply) freshly extracted coconut milk from a ripe coconut frequently.

✤ Thinning of hair : Bathe the hair in 1 teacup coconut milk twice or thrice a week for a few months. (*Note*: Avoid soap or shampoo.)

: Grind $1/2$ teacup each curry leaves, rind of chebulic myrobalan and liquorice sticks into a fine paste. Boil this in 2 teacups coconut oil till the solid mass chars. Filter and use as a hair oil.

✤ Toothache : Heat 1 tsp coconut oil and fry 3 pieces of clove. Powder. Apply on the affected area.

✤ Swelling of testicles (Orchitis) : Heat 1 tsp castor oil. Fry grated coconut obtained from one half of a mature coconut fruit and 1 tsp crushed garlic till they become brown. Remove from the fire and eat when bearably hot.

❧ Breathing problems : Mix 1 tsp camphor in $1/2$ teacup slightly warmed coconut oil and apply on the chest.

❧ Boils : Dissolve 1 tbsp refined flour in a very little water. Heat 1 tsp coconut oil and fry the flour till it is softened. Spread it over a thin muslin cloth and apply on the boil when it is still bearably warm.

❧ Prickly heat : Grind well 1 tbsp grated coconut along with 1 tsp cumin into a very fine paste. Extract the milk from this and apply on the affected area.

❧ Shoe bite : Remove a mature green leaf from the coconut tree and burn it. Mix the ash with adequate quantity of coconut oil and apply on the affected areas.

❧ Skin ailments : Mix oil cake of coconut with an equal quantity of black cumin and apply on the affected parts.

❧ To improve complexion : Mix $1/2$ tsp each wheat flour and milk cream along with the paste of 10 soaked almonds. Add 1 tsp coconut oil and apply regularly.

✤ Wrinkles : Apply coconut oil on the portions of skin and face where wrinkles set in and gently massage every night at bed time.

✤ Intestinal parasites, : To prevent such infections, add more smallpox coconuts to the daily diet.

Note: Individual results may vary.

A word of Caution

Women may avoid frequent body massage with coconut oil as it promotes abundant hair growth.

In Science

Bolton, E. R. 1928. *Oils, Fats and Fatty Foods.* London: J&A Churchill. (The uses of coconut oil.)

Copeland, E. B. 1931. *The Coconut.* London: Macmillan & Co.

Gregory, T. C. 1942. *Condensed Chemical Dictionary.* New York: Reinhold Publishing Corporation. (Chemical constituents of coconut.)

Hunter, H. and H. M. Leake. 1933. *Recent Advances in Agriculture and Plant Breeding.* London: J&A Churchill. (Scientific research on coconut.)

Jamieson, G. S. 1943. *Vegetable Fats and Oils.* New York: Reinhold Publishing Corporation. (Coconut oil and its use.)

Lim-Sylianco, C. Y. et al. 1992. Anti-genotoxic effects of coconut meal, coconut milk and coconut water. *Philippine J. Sci.* 121(3):231–235.

Nair, P. K. S. et al. 1987. Therapeutic effect of coconut shell extract in Dermatophytosis. *J. Res. Ayur. Sid.* VIII, 1&2:46–52. (Coconut exhibits a very significant anti-fungal activity.)

Patel, J. S. 1938. *The Coconut: A Monograph.* Madras: Government Press.

Coriander

Coriandrum sativum

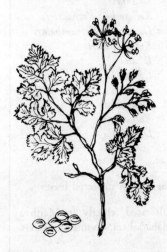

Make yours the seeds of coriander, for it is a cure for all diseases except swelling (cancer)—and that's a fatal disease.

—Prophet Muhammad (S.A.W.S.)

Cooling Mediterranean Herb

The coriander traces its origin to the Mediterranean region. It is a popular herb, well-known for its carminative and cooling properties.

Both the leaves of the coriander and its seeds find a place in the spice cupboard and also in the medicine chest.

A Useful Household Remedy

It is an effective household remedy for many *pitta* disorders, particularly those of the digestive or urinary tracts. The fresh juice of leaves can be used either internally or externally for allergies, skin rashes, itch, inflammation, etc. It facilitates digestion and absorption and is useful in the treatment of diarrhoea and dysentery.

The Profile

Botanical Name	:	*Coriandrum sativum* L.
English Names	:	Coriander, Cilantro.

Indian Names :

Bengali	: *Dhane, Dhania*
Gujarati	: *Kothmiri, Libdhana*
Hindi	: *Dhania*
Kannada	: *Kothambri, Kothamiri*
Kashmiri	: *Daaniwal, Kothambalari*
Malayalam	: *Kothumpalari*
Marathi	: *Dhana*
Oriya and Punjabi	: *Dhania*
Sanskrit	: *Dhanyaka*
Tamil	: *Kothamalli*
Telugu	: *Dhaniyalu*

Family	:	Umbelliferae.
Appearance	:	Aromatic herb with dissected leaves.
Distribution	:	Widely cultivated, chiefly in Madhya Pradesh, Maharashtra, Mysore and Bihar.
Medicinal Parts	:	Leaves, fruits.
Preparation and Dosage	:	*Infusion:* 2 tsp dried seeds steeped in 1 cup water. *Dosage:* 1 cup a day. *Powder:* Take 1/4 to 1/2 tsp at a time.

In Tradition

AILMENT   PRESCRIPTION

❧ Swellings : Drink coriander tea (1 tsp coriander seeds steeped in a cup of warm water). In addition, external application of a mixture of 2 parts turmeric powder and 1 part salt on the affected area is advised.

❧ Giddiness due to blood pressure
: Soak in a glass of water 1 tsp each coriander seeds, sandal paste and dried amla fruits. Strain it and drink the water next morning.

❧ High cholesterol
: Regular intake of coriander decoction made by boiling 2 tsp dry seed powder in 1 teacup water. (Milk and sugar can be added to improve its taste. This could be a welcome substitute for tea or coffee.) *Note:* This also acts as a diuretic as kidneys are stimulated.

❧ Abdominal pain
: Make a paste of equal quantities of dry coriander seeds, ginger and grated coconut. Add a little salt to improve its taste. Eat with rice or plain chapati.

❧ Diarrhoea
: 2 or 3 tsp coriander seeds soaked overnight in water and taken next morning with 1 teacup buttermilk.

: Boil 1 tsp cumin seeds in a cup of water. Add to this 1 tsp fresh juice of coriander leaves and a pinch of salt. Drink twice daily after meals.

❧ Dysentery, hepatitis, indigestion, nausea, typhoid fever
: 1 to 2 tsp fresh juice of coriander leaves is mixed in 1 teacup buttermilk and taken 2–3 times.

❧ Haemorrhoids : Grind $1/2$ tsp each coriander leaves and red clay into a fine paste and apply to anus.

❧ Bleeding in nose, body heat : Juice of fresh coriander leaves used as nasal drops.

❧ Burning and swelling caused due to conjunctivitis : Decoction of dried coriander powder (1 tsp seeds boiled in 1 teacup water) applied on affected parts.

❧ Cataract : Mix 1 tsp each coriander seed powder and aniseed powder. Add 2 tsp unrefined sugar. Take this mixture in the morning as well as in the evening.

❧ Headache : Mix equal quantities of sandal paste and coriander seed powder in an adequate quantity of water. Apply the paste on the affected areas.

: Extract fresh juice from coriander leaves and apply on the affected areas.

❧ Ulcer in mouth : Coriander decoction prepared by boiling 1 tsp seeds in 1 teacup water, gargled when lukewarm, frequently.

❧ Excessive menstrual flow : Boil 1 tsp coriander seeds in 2 teacups water till it is reduced to 1 teacup. Add sugar to taste and drink when lukewarm. Repeat twice or thrice a day.

❧ Blackheads, pimples : Mix 1 tsp each turmeric paste and juice of fresh coriander leaves and apply

78

daily as a face pack before going to sleep. (Also avoid fatty foods, soap, etc.)

❧ Rashes on the skin
: Apply coriander leaf paste on the affected area. Also drink coriander tea (1 tsp coriander seeds boiled in 1 cup of water).

❧ Sting and insect bites
: Drink 2 or 3 tsp coriander leaf juice mixed in 1 teacup water. Also apply sandalwood paste on the affected area.

❧ Anaemia, indigestion, kidney problems, nervous weakness, night blindness, osteoporosis, etc
: Frequent intake of coriander tea: boil or steep 2 tsp coriander powder in a glass of water. Add sugar and milk to taste.

❧ Bedwetting
: Fry 1 tsp coriander seeds in a cast iron skillet until red. Mix in 1 tsp pomegranate flowers, 1 tsp ground sesame seeds and 1 tsp gum acacia and make a fine powder. Add powdered brown sugar to equal the total amount of the powdered herbs and store. Take 1 tsp at bedtime.

❧ Fatigue
: Fry in 1 tbsp ghee $1/2$ tsp each coriander seeds, cumin seeds, black pepper, tail pepper and tuvar dal. Make a tasty rasam by adding 1 tsp rasam powder, one tomato and 1 teacup water. Drink it as an appetizer or eat with steamed rice.

♦ Vertigo   : Steep 1 tsp each dried amla powder
                             and coriander seeds in water overnight.
                             Strain and drink next morning. To
                             improve the flavour, sugar can be
                             added. Repeat for a few days.

   Note: Individual results may vary.

A Word of Caution

Coriander oil is known to cause contact dermatitis.

In Science

Dhew. 1974. *A Barefoot Doctor's Manual*. Publn. No. (NIH) 75–695.
    Washington D. C. (How coriander can be used as a household remedy.)

Farnsworth, N. R. and A. B. Segelman. 1971. Hypoglcaemic plants.
    Tile and Till 57(3):52–56. (Coriander's role in diabetes.)

Joshi, B. S. et al. 1967. Variation and covariation in some Umbelliferous
    spice crops, I. Variability in coriander. *Indian Journal of Genetics
    and Plant Breeding* Vol. 27 No. 2 pp. 211–19.

Lewis, W. H. and M. P. F. Elvin-Lewis. 1977. *Medical Botany: Plants
    Affecting Man's Health*. New York: John Wiley & Sons.

Ministry of Food and Agriculture, Farm Information Unit, Govt. of
    India. 1970. Grow Coriander for Good Profits. New Delhi. *Spice
    Pamphlet* No. 3 pp. 1–70.

Shankaracharya, N. B. and C. P. Natarajan. 1971. Coriander
    Chemistry, Technology and Uses. *Indian Spices* Vol. 8(2) p. 4.

Toghrol, F. and M. Pourebrahimi. 1976. Estimation of Vitamin C in
    fenugreek, coriander and ribes in Iran. *Plant Foods Man*. 2:1–5. (A
    chemical analysis of coriander in Iran.)

Tripathi, S. N. and C. M. Tripathi. 1992. Clinical and Experimental
    Evaluation of Endocrine Response of Herbal Drugs. *Jour. Res. Ayur.
    Sid*. XIII, 3–4:174–178. (Role of coriander as a drug.)

12

Saffron

Crocus sativus

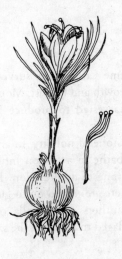

The perfumes of saffron are of very high grade.

—Brahma Vaivarta Purana
8th Century A.D.

The Chinese Connection

Commercial saffron consists of the tiny, dried stigmas and styles of the flowers. It has been known to the Chinese from time immemorial and has been greatly exploited for medical use by their barefoot doctors.

Hippocrates and other ancient authors have also written prodigiously about saffron in their treatises.

In India, compared to the Ayurvedic system, the Unani system seems to have exploited this delicate herb in a more elaborate way.

Saffron in Folklore

Saffron is used to counteract spasmodic disorders and in the treatment of several digestive disorders, particularly flatulent colic. It is useful in treating skin ailments, fevers, melancholia and enlargement of the liver and spleen, urinary and uterine troubles. A paste is often used as a dressing for sores and bruises. It is reported to improve eyesight as well, thanks to the presence of selenium.

Why Is It So Expensive?

The herb is delicate, needing extreme care for its survival. It requires specialized attention for its growth and harvest. Moreover, some 50,000 flowers need to be harvested to produce just a handful of saffron.

Saffron has often been the touchstone of nobility. In ancient Rome, aristocratic women used to bathe in a saffron infusion.

Being highly priced, saffron is prone to adulteration. Herbs such as safflower, calendula, lyperia, etc are passed on to gullible customers as saffron. Sometimes, anthers and corolla of the mother plant crocus itself are camouflaged to look like the saffron of commerce.

The Profile

Botanical Name	:	*Crocus sativus* L.	
English Names	:	Spanish Saffron, Autumn Crocus.	
Indian Names	:	Bengali	: *Jaffran*
		Gujarati	
		& Marathi	: *Keshar*
		Hindi, Punjabi	
		& Urdu	: *Zafran*

Kannada	: *Kunkuma Kesari*
Kashmiri	: *Kong*
Sanskrit	: *Kesara, Kunkuma*
Tamil	: *Kungumappoo*
Telugu	: *Kunkuma Puva*

Family	: Iridaceae.
Appearance	: A bulbous perennial.
Distribution	: Cultivated in Kashmir, Bhersar and Chaubattia in Uttar Pradesh.
Useful Parts	: The dried stigmas and tops of the styles.
Preparation and Dosage	: *Infusion*: Steep 6 to 10 stigmas in 1/2 cup water. Take 1/2 to 1 cup a day, unsweetened, a mouthful at a time.

In Tradition

AILMENT	PRESCRIPTION
❧ Diabetes	: A pinch of saffron pounded with 1/2 tsp ghee taken regularly.
❧ Internal bleeding	: Add a pinch of saffron and 1/2 tsp turmeric powder to a cup of hot milk and drink.
❧ Colic, insomnia, gas in stomach, whooping cough	: Take infusion (see above).
❧ Urine retention	: Soak a little saffron overnight in 1/4 cup water. Next morning drink it with 1 tsp honey.

83

❧ Fevers and melan-
cholia; also helps
in purification of
blood, liver or
spleen malfunc-
tioning

: Regular intake of a pinch of saffron.

❧ Baldness,
not due to
heredity

: Grind 1 tbsp liquorice root along with
1 tbsp milk and a pinch of saffron
into a fine paste. Apply this paste on
bald patches before going to bed for a
few weeks.

❧ For an easy
delivery. (*Cau-
tion:* Large doses
to be avoided by
pregnant women
as it may cause
abortion.)

: Mix a pinch of saffron with $1/2$ teacup
milk and take daily. (This can be
folded into a betel leaf and eaten as
well.)

❧ Menstrual pains,
lumbar pain acco-
mpanying men-
struation, hysteria,
leucorhhoea

: Boil 1 tsp saffron in $1/4$ teacup water.
Let it reduce to become 1 tbsp. Divide
this decoction into three portions and
take with equal quantity of water, thrice
daily for a couple of days.

❧ Sexual debility

: Mix $1/8$ tsp saffron with milk. Take
twice daily.

: Take a pinch of saffron wrapped in a
betel leaf or with almonds.

❧ Cold and phlegm
in children

: Grind $1/2$ tsp saffron in milk (pre-
ferably human milk) and apply on
nose, head, cheeks, etc.

84

✤ For complexion
   improvement and
   freshness of
   face

: Mix 2 tbsp almonds, 2 tbsp semolina
and 2 tsp saffron and make a fine
powder. Mix this powder with a little
cow's milk so as to make small tablets
the size of chick-peas. Once dry, these
can be stored. Use a tablet after mixing
with cream and massage over face. Soap
is to be avoided.

✤ For complexion
   improvement

: Add a pinch of saffron to 1 tbsp milk
and take on an empty stomach every
morning.

Note: Individual results may very.

A Word of Caution

Saffron is reported to contain a poison that acts on the Central
Nervous System and damages the kidneys when taken in excess.

Large doses of saffron could prove fatal: 2 full tsp and above
is considered a fatal dose for human beings.

In Science

Atal, C. K. 1982. Saffron in Kashmir. *Proc. Symp. Flavours & their
Industrial Applications.* Jammu. 52–55. (Uses of saffron.)

Chopra, R. N. et al. 1969. *Glossary of Indian Medicinal Plants.* New
Delhi: Council of Scientific and Industrial Research. (A brief account
of saffron.)

De, Amit Krishna. 1995. Saffron. *Spice India* 8:10.

Mandan, C. L. et al. 1966. Saffron. *Econ. Bot.* 20(4):377–385.
(Usefulness of saffron.)

Sastry, L. V. L. et al. 1955. Saffron (*Crocus sativus* Linn). *J. Sci. Industr. Res.* 14A(44):178–184. (An introduction.)

Srivastava, G. S. 1958. Growing saffron in Lucknow. *J. Bombay Nat. Hist. Soc.* 55:385–386. (Horticultural aspects.)

Srivastava, T. N. et al. 1985. Important Medicinal Plants of Jammu and Kashmir I—*Kesar* (Saffron). *Ancient Sci. Life* 5(1): 68–73.

13

Cumin
Cuminum cyminum

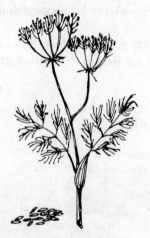

Grind cumin seeds with a drop of ghee and a pinch of salt. Apply for scorpion sting.

—Charaka Samhita

Biblical Remedy

Cumin has been well-known for its carminative action since Biblical times. Iran is the major exporter of cumin. The chief trading centres for cumin in India are: Jabalpur, Ratlam, Jaipur and Gangapur.

Cumin Fruits—and Not Cumin Seeds!

Although loosely referred to as seeds, cumin consists really of fruits. They are stomachic, antispasmodic, astringent, carminative, sedative and stimulant and are useful in diarrhoea and dyspepsia. They help in relieving nausea, particularly in the case of pregnant women.

Cumin in Cuisine

In Holland and Switzerland, cumin is used to season certain cheese varieties. In France and Germany it is used to flavour bread and pastries. It is also employed in several native dishes of South America. Back in India, it is sprinkled everywhere, on almost everything: a dash of cumin finds its place in every conceivable dish or curry powder; anything made of cereals, vegetables, meat, fruits, or yoghurt is bound to have a sprinkling of cumin.

It is believed in Ayurveda that cumin has a cooling effect on the human body and therefore it has a definitive role particularly in warm seasons and climates.

The Profile

Botanical Names	:	*Cuminum cyminum* L. *Cuminum odorum* Salisb.
Indian Names	:	Bengali, Hindi,
		Oriya & Punjabi : *Jeera*
		Gujarati : *Jiru, Jeeru*
		Kannada : *Jeerige*
		Kashmiri : *Zyur*
		Malayalam : *Jirakam*
		Marathi : *Jeregire*
		Sanskrit : *Jiraka*
		Sindhi : *Zero*
		Tamil : *Seeragam*
		Telugu : *Jidakara, Jikaka*
Family	:	Umbelliferae.
Appearance	:	A slender annual herb with angular striated stem bearing two or three partite linear bluish-green leaves. Flowers white

or rose, in umbels. Fruits greyish, about
$1/4$ inch long, tapering towards both ends.
Seeds yellowish to greyish brown in
colour, when dried.

Distribution   : Cultivated in almost all states with the
exception of Bengal and Assam. Uttar
Pradesh and Punjab are the major
producers.

Medicinal Parts   : Fruits, often referred to as seeds.

In Tradition

AILMENT	PRESCRIPTION
❧ Diabetes	: Crush 8 tsp cumin into a fine powder. Take $1/2$ tsp with water twice daily.
❧ High blood pressure	: Mix 1 tsp finely ground cumin powder in 2 tbsp each coconut water and milk and $1/4$ tsp freshly ground sandal paste and sugar to taste. Drink this mixture every morning for a few days.
❧ Constipation, indigestion	: Add equal quantities of cumin seeds, pepper and dried ginger to a bunch of dried curry leaves and powder them together. Add a little salt to taste. Add this mixture to hot ghee and eat along with steamed rice.
❧ Diarrhoea	: Combine 1 tsp each of the powders of cumin, ginger, cinnamon and honey and mix into a thick paste. Take $1/2$ to 1 tsp thrice daily.

❧ Diarrhoea, digestive disorder
: Boil 1 tsp cumin seeds in a glass of water. Add to this 1 tsp fresh juice of coriander leaves and a pinch of salt. Drink twice daily after meals for 2–3 days.

❧ Gas
: Mix equal quantities of broken cumin, black pepper and ginger. Make an infusion by mixing in some warm water. Drink twice or thrice a day for a few days.

❧ Giddiness, indigestion, nausea
: Soak cumin seeds in lime juice overnight. Dry them in the sun and bottle. Chew $1/2$ tsp of this mixture along with a glass of warm water after food for a few days.

❧ Heaviness in stomach, indigestion
: Mix $1/4$ tsp each powdered cumin and pepper in a glass of buttermilk. Drink two or three times a day for 2–3 days.

❧ To increase lactation
: Mix together 1 tsp each cumin powder and sugar and take with warm milk after dinner every day for a few days.

: Boil 2 tsp cumin in $1/2$ cup water. Filter. Mix in $1/2$ cup milk and 1 tsp honey. Drink once a day for a few days.

❧ Prickly heat
: Grind 1 tbsp cumin with coconut milk and apply frequently.

❧ Scorpion bite
: Grind 1 tsp cumin with juice of one onion and apply.

❧ Body heat, nausea, *pitta-*aggravation
: Mix equal quantities of powdered cumin, pepper, dried ginger and the rind of pomegranate fruit. Fry them in a little ghee and take with cooked rice twice or thrice a day for three days.

❧ Fatigue
: Mix 1/2 tsp each broken cumin, coriander seeds, black pepper, long pepper and tuvar dal. Boil in water and drink with salt to taste.

❧ Insomnia
: Mix 1 tsp powder of fried cumin with a mashed ripe banana. Eat at night' regularly.

❧ *Pitta-*aggravation
: Mix 2 tbsp cumin in 3 teacups gingelly oil. Massage the head once a week before washing.

Note: Individual results may vary.

In Science

Chandola, R. P. et al. 1970. Cumin cultivation in Rajasthan. *Indian Farming* 20(4). p. 13. (Horticultural aspects of cumin.)

Debray, M. et al. 1971. *Contribution a l'inventaire des plantes medicinales de Madagascar.* (Travaux et documents de l'O.R.S.T.O.M., no. 8) Paris. (Cumin in Madagascar.) (In French)

Farnsworth, N. R. et al. 1975. Potential value of plants as sources of new antifertility agents, II. *J. Pharm. Sci.* 64(5):715–754. (Cumin is one of the dependable sources of new antifertility agents.)

Hartwell, J. L. 1971. Plants used against cancer—A survey. *Lloydia* 34:386–425. (Cumin's role in fighting cancer.)

Ministry of Food & Agriculture, Govt. of India. 1971. *Cumin*. New Delhi: Farm Information Unit, Dte. of Extension.

Opdyke, D. L. J. 1974. Monograph on fragrance, raw materials. *Food Cosmet. Toxicol.* 12 (Suppl.):807–1016. (Phototoxic effects reported from undiluted cumin oil.)

Ramadan, F. M. et al. 1972. Anti-bacterial effects of some essential oils. I: Use of agar-diffusion method. *Chem. Mikrobiol. Technol. Lebensm* 2:51–55; *Chem. Abstr.* 77:122532. (How cumin oil fights bacteria.) (In German)

Rockwell, P. and I. Raw. 1979. A mutagenic screening of various herbs, spices and food additives. *Nutr. Cancer 1(4):10–15.*

Shankaracharya, N. B. and C. P. Natarajan. 1971. Chemical composition and uses of cumin. *Indian Food Packer* 25(6):22–28. (Cumin, its chemical architecture and its functional competence.)

Sievers, A. F. 1948. Production of drug and condiment plants. *U.S. Dep. Agric. Farmers' Bull.* 1999. 99. (Cumin cultivation.)

Tassan, C. G. and G. F. Russell. 1975. Chemical and sensory studies of cumin. *J. Food Sci.* 40:1185–1188. (The odour of cumin is attributed to the aldehydes present in the oil.)

Toghrol, F. and H. Daneshpejouh. 1974. Estimation of free aminoacids, protein and aminoacid compositions of cumin seed (*Cuminum cyminum*) of Iran *J. Trop. Pediatr. Environ. Child Health* 20:109–111. (Cumin and its chemical profile.)

14

Turmeric

Curcuma longa

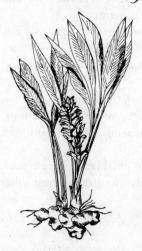

*All poisons can be removed
from the human body if
treated with a paste of
turmeric.*

—Matsya Purana
218, 20. (8th Century A.D.)

Finest Indian Turmeric!

India is the single largest producer of turmeric in the world. Over two lakh tonnes is grown for home consumption and export every year.

There are as many as 16 identified varieties of turmeric, of which Alleppey Turmeric is considered to be the best. Rating is done mainly on the basis of the richness of the colouring matter.

Turmeric, the Therapeutic

Turmeric is a herb indispensable in Hindu traditions and rituals. In the southern parts of India housewives exchange the rootstock on festive occasions. It is an important ingredient in Indian cuisine and cosmetics.

As several parts of India are tropical or sub-tropical, there is a constant invasion of germs, virus, bacteria and fungi. This results in high rates of bio-degradability. It is here that turmeric comes into its own. Mere sprinkling of turmeric powder in every dish—as is being done by Indian housewives and cooks—provides protection against innumerable tropical germs.

Turmeric is an ideal disinfectant and scouring agent. It acts as an internal antiseptic. It cools down the digestive, circulatory and reproductive systems, arrests cholesterol problems and eliminates toxins.

It is found useful by patients suffering from diabetes, leprosy, ulcer, impotency, gallstones, jaundice, respiratory wounds, inflammation, rheumatism, arthritis, anaemia, stiffness of limbs, etc.

With herbs such as fenugreek, cumin, black pepper, tulsi, etc, turmeric assumes synergy in combating bacteria and other pathogens.

The Physician's Choice

The turmeric which is available commercially for cooking purposes is the boiled, debarked rootstock which, in processing, has lost many of its miraculous medicinal properties. The raw, dried rootstocks of the plant are therefore preferred by discerning native physicians.

The Profile

Botanical Names	:	*Curcuma longa* L.
		(*Curcuma domestica* Val).
English Name	:	Turmeric.

Indian Names	:	Bengali	: *Halud, Pitras*
		Gujarati	: *Haldi, Haldhar*
		Hindi	: *Haldi*
		Kannada	: *Arishina*
		Konkani	: *Halad*
		Malayalam	: *Manjal, Haridra*
		Marathi	: *Halede, Halad*
		Oriya	: *Haldi*
		Punjabi	: *Haldar, Haldi*
		Sanskrit	: *Haladi, Haridra, Harita*
		Tamil	: *Manjal*
		Telugu	: *Pasupu*
		Urdu	: *Haladi*

Family	:	Zingiberaceae.
Appearance	:	The spice turmeric consists of the dried, boiled, cleaned and polished rootstock of the plant. The plant has a large tuft of leaves and spikes with pale green flowering bracts, covering yellow flowers.
Distribution	:	Andhra Pradesh, Orissa, Maharashtra, Tamil Nadu, Karnataka and Kerala grow the bulk.
Medicinal Parts	:	Rootstock (rhizome), referred to as root.

In Tradition

AILMENT	PRESCRIPTION
❧ Muscle strain	: Heat ginger paste with turmeric paste (1:1) and apply.
❧ Swelling	: Mix 2 tsp turmeric powder and 1 tsp salt and apply.

95

❧ Anaemia : Take 1 tsp each raw turmeric juice and honey mixed together every morning.

❧ Bleeding (internal) : Mix 1/2 tsp turmeric and a pinch of saffron in 1 teacup warm milk and drink.

❧ Cholera, dysentery, indigestion, skin infections, body heat : Soak 1 tbsp turmeric bits in slaked lime for a couple of hours. Remove the bits. Dry them in the sun. Powder them. This rose-coloured powder can be preserved in a vial. Ten pinches of this powder are to be taken along with hot water, milk or honey. Twice daily.

❧ Intestinal worms : Take 1 tsp raw turmeric juice, mixed with a pinch of salt first thing in the morning.

❧ Jaundice : Take 1/4 tsp turmeric along with a glass of hot water 2 or 3 times daily.

❧ Common cold and sore throat : Add 1 tbsp turmeric powder to boiling water. Inhale the vapours.

❧ Dental problems and gum diseases : Turmeric, burnt, and finely powdered, used as toothpowder.

❧ Eye diseases : Boil 1 tsp turmeric powder thoroughly in 2 teacups water till it is reduced to 1 teacup. Allow to cool. A few drops of this cold infusion is used as eye drops.

❧ Ophthalmia

: Juice extracted from turmeric rhizomes, used as eye drops.

❧ Dry cough and throat infection

: Add ¹/₄ tsp turmeric powder to hot cow's milk. Drink in the morning.

❧ Asthma, dry cough, throat infection

: A glass of milk is poured on a hot ladle with a teaspoonful of turmeric powder in it and boiled over a slow fire.

❧ Common cold

: Mix 1 tsp turmeric powder along with ¹/₄ tsp ajwain powder in 3 teacups hot water. Allow to cool. Take 1 tbsp of this decoction along with 1 tsp honey twice daily for a few days.

❧ Acne

: Mix ¹/₂ tsp each turmeric and sandal powder in 1 tsp water and apply.

❧ Boils

: Apply a paste of ¹/₂ tsp each turmeric and ginger powder.

: Take 2 tsp latex (milk) of calotropis and add 1 tsp turmeric powder. Mix thoroughly and apply. Repeat.

: Slightly roast a big onion on a naked flame. Mash it and mix in 1 tsp each turmeric powder and ghee. Apply and tie a bandage.

❧ Wounds, boils, tropical skin diseases, etc

: Fine paste of turmeric applied on the affected areas.

❧ Burns : Make a paste of 1 tsp fresh gel of aloe with 1 tsp turmeric powder and apply.

❧ Corn on the foot : Finely grind 1 tsp each turmeric, calamus and henna leaves and apply on the soles.

❧ Cracks in the sole, itch, skin infections : Finely grind equal quantities of turmeric and neem leaves and apply on the affected areas.

❧ Dull and lifeless skin : Mix equal quantities of the flour of green gram, besan and turmeric powder. Use as a substitute for soap.

❧ Unwanted hair and dull complexion : Apply a fine paste of turmeric on the skin frequently.

❧ Eczema and other parasitic skin diseases, itching, smallpox, ringworm : Grind 1 tbsp each turmeric, neem leaves and gingelly oil into a fine paste; apply on the affected parts.

❧ Skin infections : Apply the juice of raw turmeric rhizomes on the affected parts.

❧ Skin infection in between the toes : Grind equal quantities of turmeric and chebulic myrobalan and apply the paste in between the toes.

❧ Whitlow : Mix turmeric powder with a little slaked lime (*chuna*) and apply.

❧ Wounds : Grind a piece of chebulic myrobalan with turmeric and neem leaves (equal

quantities). Add a little lime juice and
make a paste. Apply.

🍂 Pain (external)   : Mix 2 tsp ginger paste with 1 tsp
turmeric and warm and spread over a
cotton cloth. Place it on the affected
area and apply a bandage over it.

Note: Individual results may vary.

A Word of Caution

As the antifertility properties of turmeric have been scientifically
proved, those who desire children may avoid its excessive use.

Excess intake of turmeric is not recommended, as it is found
to cause toxicity in certain cases.

In Science

Banerjee, A. and S. S. Nigam. 1978. Anti-fungal efficacy of the essential
oils derived from various species of the genus *Curcuma* Linn. *J. Res.
Indian Med. Yoga and Homoeo.* 13(2):63–70. (Turmeric as a fungicide.)

Bhatia, A. et al. 1964. Effect of curcumin, its alkali salts and *Curcuma
longa* oil in histamine-induced gastric ulceration. *Indian J. Exp.
Biol.* 2:158–160. (Turmeric can cure ulcers.)

Bhavani Sankar, T. N. and V. Srinivasamurthy. 1979. Effect of turmeric
(*Curcuma longa*) fractions on the growth of some intestinal and
pathogenic bacteria *in vitro. Indian J. Exptl. Biol.* 17(12):1363–1366.
(Turmeric as antiseptic.)

Chopra, R. N. et al. 1956. *Glossary of Indian Medicinal Plants.* New
Delhi: Council of Scientific and Industrial Research. 85. (Antiseptic
and anti-bacterial properties in the rhizome.)

Deodhar, S. D. et al. 1980. Preliminary study on antirheumatic activity of curcumin (diferuloyl methane). *Indian J. Med. Res.* 71:632–634 (Anti-inflammatory and anti-arthritic acivities of curcumin, the active principle in turmeric.)

Dinesh Chandra and S. S. Gupta. 1972. Anti-inflammatory and anti-arthritic activity of volatile oil of *Curcuma longa* (haldi). *Indian J. Med. Res.* 60(1):138–142. (The protective effect of turmeric's essential oil in early inflammatory lesions was attributed to the anti-histaminic property.)

Ghatak, N. and N. Basu. 1972. Sodium curcuminate as an effective anti-inflammatory agent. *Indian J. Exp. Biol.* 10:235–236.

Gupta, B. et al. 1980. Mechanism of curcumin-induced gastric ulcers in rats. *Indian J. Med. Res.* 71:806–814. (Marked reduction in mucin content appeared to be the reason for ulcerogenicity of curcumin.)

Huhtanen, C. N. 1980. Inhibition of *Clostridium botulinum* by spice extracts and aliphatic alcohols. *J. Food Prod.* 43(3):195–196; *Chem. Abstr.* 92, 209491e, 1980. (Antiseptic and anti-bacterial properties of turmeric.)

Garg, S. K. et al. 1978. Screening of Indian plants for antifertility activity. *Indian J. Exptl. Biol.* 16(10):1077–1079. (Antifertility activity of turmeric.)

Iyengar, M. A. et al. 1995. Anti-microbial activity of the essential oil of *Curcuma longa* leaves. *Indian Drugs* 32(6):249–250. (Activity of essential oil against gram-negative bacteria and pathogenic fungus even at 1:32 dilutions significant.)

Jain, J. P. et al. 1979. Clinical trials of *Haridra (Curcuma longa)* in cases of *Tamak Swasa* and *Kasa. J. Res. Indian Med. Yoga & Homoeo.* 14(2):110–120. (Turmeric effective against cough and dyspnoea.)

Jain, J. P. et al. 1990. A clinical trial of volatile oil of *Curcuma longa* Linn. (*Haridra*) in cases of bronchial asthma (*Tamaka Swasa*). *Jour. Res. Ayur. Sid.* XI, 1–4:20–30. (Efficacy of turmeric in bronchial asthma.)

Janaki, N. and T. R. Ingle. 1967. An improved method for the isolation of Curcumin from turmeric (*Curcuma longa* L.). *J. Indian Chem. Soc. 44:985.* (An efficient extraction method reported.)

Keshavarz, K. 1976. Influence of turmeric and curcumin on cholesterol concentration of eggs and tissues. *Poult. Sci.* 55(3):1077–1083. (Turmeric can bring down cholesterol levels.)

Kiso, Y. et al. 1983. Validity of Oriental Medicines, Part 53. Liver-protecting drugs, Part 8. Antihepatotoxic principles of *Curcuma longa rhizome. Planta Med.* 49(3):185–187. (The liver-protector in the rhizome.)

Kuttan, R. et al. 1987. Turmeric and Curcumin as topical agents in cancer therapy. *Tumori* 73(1):29–31. (Role of turmeric against cancer.)

Kositchaiwat, C. et al. 1993. *Curcuma longa* Linn. in the treatment of gastric ulcer—Comparison to liquid antacid: a controlled clinical trial. *J. Med. Assoc. Thai.* 76(11): 601–605. (Turmeric is efficacious in treating gastric ulcers.)

Lutomski, J. et al. 1974. Effect of an alcohol extract and active ingredients from *Curcuma longa* on bacteria and fungi. *Planta Med.* 26(1):9–19. (Anti-bacterial and anti-fungal properties of turmeric.)

Mukerji, B. et al. 1961. Spices and gastric function. Part I—Effect of *Curcuma longa* on the gastric secretion in rabbits. *J. Sci. Industr. Res.* 20C:25–28. (Utility of turmeric in gastric functions.)

Pachauri, S. P. and S. K. Mukherjee. 1970. Effect of *Curcuma longa* (*Haridra*) and *Curcuma amada* (*Amragandhi*) on the cholesterol level in experimental hypercholesterolaemia of rabbits. *J. Res. Indian Med.* 5:27–31. (Effects of turmeric on the cholesterol level.)

Rao, T. S. et al. 1982. Anti-inflammatory activity of Curcumin analogues. *Indian J. Med. Res.* 75:574–578. (Anti-inflammatory and anti-arthritic effects of turmeric.)

Sankar, T. N. B. et al. 1980. Toxicity studies on turmeric (*Curcuma longa*). Acute toxicity studies in rats, guineapigs and monkeys. *Indian J. Exptl. Biol.* 18(1):73–75. (Toxicity of turmeric.)

Sethi, S. C. and J. S. Agarwal. 1952. Stabilization of Edible Fats by Spices and Condiments. Part I. *J. Sci. Industr. Res. 11B:46.* (Turmeric checks the development of rancidity in vegetable oils.)

Sinha, M. et al. 1976. Studies on the effects of *Curcuma longa* on aspirin-induced gastric lesions. *Nagarjun* 19(6):11–12. (Protection against gastric lesions.)

Soni, K. B. et al. Reversal of aflatoxin-induced liver damage by turmeric and curcumin. *Cancer Lett.* 66(2):115–121. (Action on liver.)

Srihari Rao, T. et al. 1982. Anti-inflammatory activity of *Curcuma* analogues. *Indian J. Med. Res.* 75:574–578. (A commentary on the anti-inflammatory activity of turmeric.)

Srinivas, C. and K. V. S. Prabhakar. 1987. Clinical, bacteriological study of *Curcuma longa* on conjunctivitis. *Antiseptic* 84(3):166–168. (Turmeric can cure conjunctivitis, control the growth of *E. coli* and *Staphylococcus aureus* very effectively.)

Srivastava, R. et al. 1985. Anti-thrombolytic effect of Curcumin. *Thrombosis Res.* 40:413–417.

Subba Rao, D. et al. 1970. Effect of curcumin on serum and liver cholesterol levels in the rat. *J. Nutr.* 100:1307–1315.

Thakur, D. K. et al. 1983. Trial of some of the plant extracts and chemicals for their anti-fungal activity in calves. *Indian Vet. J.* 60(10):799–801. (Anti-fungal activity of turmeric extracts.)

Veluchamy, G. et al. 1982. Role of Siddha medicine in the treatment of rheumatoid arthritis (*Santhi Vatha Soolai*). *Rheumatism* 17(2):68–75. (Anti-arthritic activity of turmeric.)

15

Dhatura

Datura stramonium

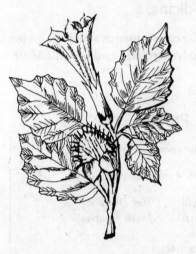

Offer flowers of Dhatura to Trilochana in the month of Shravana.

—Vamana Purana 16.32. (2nd Century A.D.)

The Herb of Shiva

Dhatura is known as *Chandrashekhara* in the ancient herbal texts of India, after its mythological association with Lord Shiva.

Dhatura and the Tradition of Medicine

Dhatura is a well-known drug in traditional medicine in India. It is widely used in poisoning due to the bites of insects and animals, particularly in the treatment of dog bite, snake bite, etc. It possesses properties analogous to those of belladonna as it counteracts spasmodic disorders and induces sleep.

Both seeds and leaves of dhatura are inhaled in whooping cough, asthma and other respiratory diseases. For the rheumatic swellings of joints, lumbago, sciatica and neuralgia, the leaf, smeared with an oil, is warmed and applied. Sometimes the leaf is made into a poultice and applied.

Dhatura in Unani Medicine

In the Unani system, *Roghan Dhatura* is used as a massage oil for the paralysed portion of the body. Seeds are used in *Haba Shafa*, a sure cure for asthma.

The Profile

Botanical Name	:	*Dhatura stramonium* L.
English Names	:	Thorn Apple, Stramonium.
Indian Names	:	Bengali : *Shet Dhatura*
		Gujarati : *Dholo Dhaturo*
		Hindi, Punjabi & Sanskrit : *Dhatura*
		Malayalam : *Ummattam, Ummam*
		Tamil : *Oomathai*
		Telugu : *Tellavummetta, Datturamu.*
Family	:	Solanaceae.
Appearance	:	A common weed. Leaves, egg-shaped, toothed, pubescent, oblique at the base of lamina. Flowers white. Fruits covered with prickles.
Distribution	:	Grows in wastelands of the country.

104

Medicinal Parts	:	Dried leaves, top portion of the flowers, seeds, root.
Other Species	:	*Dhatura metel L. (Sadahdhatura), Safed Dhatura, Kanak*. Flowers, white to yellowish, often violet coloured outside; the flowers have double corolla whorls. The leaves and seeds have similar properties like *stramonium*.
	:	*Dhatura innoxia* Mill. *(Sadahdhatura)*. The corolla is 10-angled (unlike in *D. metel*, which is 5-angled). Fruits have very slender spines and brown seeds. Properties, similar to *stramonium*.

In Tradition

AILMENT   PRESCRIPTION

✤ Swollen legs   : Mix 1/2 teacup each of the juices of dhatura leaves, madar leaves and ginger. Allow the mixture to boil in 1/2 teacup sesame oil. Cool and apply on the swollen limbs.

✤ Baldness   : Make a paste of 2 tsp each liquorice root and seeds of dhatura, a little saffron and 1 tsp milk cream. Fry this paste in 2 tsp coconut oil till charred. Apply on bald patches. (*Caution*: Dhatura is poisonous.)

             : Grind a tender fruit of dhatura and apply on the bald patches.(*Note*: Some doctors recommend that one's own saliva be used for grinding the tender fruit, instead of water.)

✤ Earache : Put a few drops of leaf juice into the affected ear.

✤ Earache, suppurative conditions of the ear : Boil 1/2 teacup each dhatura leaf juice and sesame oil in a tin vessel on a low fire. When half of the juice has evaporated, put in 7 leaves of madar, smeared with oil and sprinkled with a little salt. Boil till they are charred. Strain and bottle. Use as ear drops.

✤ Soreness in the eye : Put a few drops of leaf juice into the ear, opposite the affected eye.

✤ To stop lactation : Tie warmed leaves of dhatura on the breasts.

✤ Boils : Warm dhatura leaves. Tie on the affected areas.

: Smear a little castor oil on dhatura leaves and heat over the flame. Tie as bandage on the affected parts.

: Burn the shoots of dhatura in hot ashes. Mix the ash with an adequate quantity of castor oil and apply on the affected parts.

✤ Snakebite : Crush the roots of dhatura and mix with lime juice and tie on the bitten area.

✦ Mental   : Soak a few dhatura flowers in water
  derangement   and use this for washing the head every
                    day. (*Caution*: Dhatura is poisonous.)

Note: Individual results may vary.

A Word of Caution

Dhatura is a highly poisonous plant and hence extreme care has
to be exercised while handling it. Any treatment has to be
undertaken under the direct supervision of a medical practitioner.

The drug is for external use only.

Grind lotus root in milk and take 1 tsp thrice a day for two
days, in case dhatura poisoning is noticed.

In Science

Gupta, S. and C. L. Madan. 1972. Effect of some physical, chemical
    and hormonal treatments and ageing on the germination of *Dhatura
    metel* L. seeds. *Herba hung.* 11(2):27–31. (A study on the
    germination of dhatura seeds.)

Kapahi, B. K. and Y. K. Sarin. 1972–73. A note on the utilization of
    Dhatura stramonium Linn. occurring wild in N. W. Himalayas.
    Indian Drugs 10:11–15.

Kaul, B. L. et al. 1976. Stimulation of growth and development of
    Dhatura by low doses of radiations. *Stimulation Newslett.* 9:17–26.
    (Effect of radiation on the growth of dhatura.)

Khaleque, A. et al. 1967. Investigations of *Dhatura fastusa (D. metel)*
    II. Isolation of daturanolone and fastusic acid from the seeds.
    Pakistan J. Scient. Ind. Res. 10:85. (Minor alkaloids isolated from
    the seeds of *Dhatura metel.*)

Madan, C. L. et al. 1966. The distribution of the total alkaloids in the different organs of some Dhatura species/varieties. *Curr. Sci.* 35:311–312. (Variations in alkaloid content in different parts of the plant.)

Prabhakar, V. S. et al. 1971. Utilization of wild dhaturas of N. W. India for commercial production of hyoscine. *Indian J. Pharm.* 33:35–36.

Raffauf, R. F. 1970. *Handbook of Alkaloids and Alkaloid-containing Plants.* New York: Wiley Inter Science. (Dhatura is rich in hyoscyamine and scopolamine, the principal alkaloids.)

Sairam, T. V. and P. Khanna. 1971. Effect of Tyrosine and Phenylalanine on Growth and Production of Alkaloids in *Dhatura tatula* Tissue Cultures. *Lloydia* 34(1):170–171.

Sobti, S. N. and B. L. Kaul. 1982. Cultivation of *Dhatura innoxia* and *Dhatura metel* in India. *Cultivation and Utilization of Medicinal Plants* ed. C. K. Atal and B. M. Kapur. Jammu: CSIR. Regional Research Laboratory. 259–261. (Horticultural aspects of dhatura.)

Trease, C. E and W. C. Evans. 1983. *Pharmacognosy* 12th edn. London: Bailliere Tindall. 500.

16

Cardamom

Elettaria cardamomum

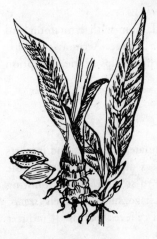

*As the prayer of Lord
Pashupati relieves a person
from the bondage of the
world, the decoction of
cardamom instantly cures the
suppression of urination.*

—Ayurveda Saukhyam of
Todaraananda

Pride of Kerela

Among the spices of India, cardamom occupies a pre-eminent
position, perhaps only next to black pepper.

It is the second largest foreign-exchange earner of India among
the spices and condiments exported. The country meets almost
sixty per cent of the global demand for cardamom. Sri Lanka,
Guatemala and Thailand are the other major producers of cardamom.

Kerala alone harvests nearly sixty per cent of the entire
cardamom production in the country.

Cardamom: Some Buying Tips

Cardamom of commerce which consists of the dried capsules,
enclosing the invaluable aromatic seeds, comes in various grades

and qualities. While the green colour of the skin is an indicator of the freshness of the crop, the real quality of cardamom lies in its seed-content. While buying cardamom, it is necessary to ensure that the seed pods are not cracked, hollow, empty, shrivelled, immature or insect-infested. The capsules should be compact and filled with seeds.

The Three Aromatics

In medicine, a combination of cardamom with cinnamon and bay leaves is referred to as The Three Aromatics. This combination is a valuable digestive which helps in the absorption of medicines.

Cardamom and Its Use

Cardamom awakens the spleen, stimulates the heart and imparts clarity and peace of mind. It possesses digestive, antispasmodic and carminative properties. It helps to stop belching, vomiting or acid regurgitation. It dissolves blockages in all channels (*srotas*) and opens up the nervous system. It relieves spasms. It induces perspiration and restores circulation.

When added to milk it neutralizes its mucus-forming properties. It also detoxifies the caffeine in coffee.

The Profile

| Botanical Names | : | *Elettaria Cardamomum* (L) Maton. Var. *minor* Watt. |
| English Names | : | Cardamom, Lesser Cardamom, Green Cardamom, Malabar Cardamom. |

110

Indian Names	:	Bengali	: *Chhoti Elaichi*
		Gujarati	: *Elaichi*
		Hindi	: *Chhoti Elaichi*
		Kannada	: *Yelakki*
		Kashmiri	: *Aa'l Budu Aa'l*
		Malayalam	: *Elathari*
		Marathi	: *Velchi*
		Oriya	: *Aliaichi*
		Sanskrit	: *Ela*
		Tamil	: *Elakkai*
		Telugu	: *Elakkaayulu*

Family	:	Zingiberaceae.
Appearance	:	A herb with fleshy branched rhizome. Leaves very large, narrow. Flowering stock arises from the base of the stem.
Distribution	:	In South India, particularly in the wet forests and hilly regions in Kerala and Karnataka. Also cultivated in Assam, Maharashtra and Tamil Nadu.
Medicinal Parts	:	Seeds.

In Tradition

AILMENT	PRESCRIPTION
❧ Giddiness due to BP	: Mix 1 tsp cardamom seeds with 2 tsp dried ginger, long pepper and liquorice. Powder it. Add 5 tbsp sugar. Take $1/2$ tsp in a cup of hot water twice a day.
❧ Absorption problems— particularly in small intestine	: Mix and finely powder equal quantities of cardamom, dried ginger and nutmeg. Take 1 tsp with warm water.

111

❧ Dyspepsia, indigestion, loss of taste, nausea, poor absorption
: Boil 1 tsp mint leaves in 1 cup water. Take off the fire. Add $1/2$ tsp powdered cardamom seeds, mix and drink (*Note:* cardamom should never be boiled).

❧ Indigestion
: Mix and finely powder equal quantities of asafoetida, dried ginger, rock salt and cardamom seeds. Take 1 tsp of this mixture along with warm water.

❧ Indigestion
: Make a fine powder of 1 tsp each cardamom and saunf seeds. Take $1/4$ tsp with water twice daily after meals.

❧ Gas in stomach
: Make an infusion of equal parts of cardamom, saunf and ginger. Take 1 tsp in 1 teacup water along with a pinch of asafoetida.

❧ Bad breath or halitosis
: Make an infusion of 1 tsp each of cardamom, cinnamon and bay leaves in 1 teacup water. Drink it. (Also, cleanse the mouth with liquorice powder and chew some saunf frequently.)

❧ Migraine, vertigo
: Heat 2 tbsp sesame oil. Mix in $1/2$ tsp each finely powdered cardamom and cinnamon. Apply on the head.

❧ Nasal congestion
: Put 1 tsp cardamom seeds on burning coal and inhale the smoke.

❧ Tooth problems
: Mix and finely powder equal quantities of liquorice, dried ginger and

cardamon seeds. Take 1 tsp of the mixture with honey.

❧ Hoarseness, pharyngitis, sore throat
: Pour 1 glass boiling water on a mixture of 1 tsp each cinnamon and cardamom. Filter and use as a gargle when warm.

❧ Blockage of nose due to severe cold
: Make into a very fine powder equal quantities of the following: cardamom seeds, cinnamon, black pepper and cumin. Sniff this powder frequently to induce sneezing.

❧ Cough and cold, eyesight weakness, hoarse voice, nervous weakness
: Mix seeds of cardamom along with 1 tbsp honey. Eat every day.

❧ Mucus in cough
: Pour 1 teacup boiling water over $1/2$ tsp each ginger powder, clove powder and cinnamon powder. Filter. Sweeten with 1 tsp honey and drink.

❧ Dry cough
: Add 2 cardamoms, 10 raisins and 5 corns of tail pepper in 1 teacup of boiling water. Sip. Repeat after 2–3 hrs.

❧ Diarrhoea, dysentery, exhaustion due to overwork, heart palpitation, scanty urination, depression
: Boil $1/4$ tsp powdered seeds in thin tea water and drink.

❧ Constipation,   : Grind a piece of preserve of chebulic
   giddiness   myrobalan (*Caution:* Seed to be
                       removed). Finely grind it along with
                       1/2 tsp coriander seeds and 1/4 tsp
                       cardamom seeds. Take this mixture
                       twice a day.

❧ Giddiness   : Boil 1/2 tsp cardamom seeds and 1 tsp
                       palmyrah sugar in 2 teacups water, till
                       the water is reduced to 1 teacup. Take
                       half a cup of this liquid twice a day.

Note: Individual results may vary.

A Word of Caution

Excessive use of cardamom is believed to cause impotency.

Patients with ulcers and high *pitta* are not advised the frequent use of cardamom.

In Science

Abraham, P. 1965. The cardamom in India. *Farm-Bulletin* (New Series) 37:1–46. (A monograph on cardamom.)

Cardamom Board. 1970. *Cardamom.* Cochin-18:1–8. (A mini-monograph on cardamom.)

Burkill, I. H. 1935. *A Dictionary of Economic Products of the Malayan Peninsula.* 2 vols. London: Crown Agents for the Colonies. (Economic uses of cardamom.)

Frawley, D and V. Lad. 1994. *The Yoga of Herbs.* Delhi. (Cardamom and its medicinal use.)

Hill, A. F. 1937. *Economic Botany.* New York: McGraw Hill. (Economic uses of cardamom.)

Jain, S. K. 1968. *Medicinal Plants.* New Delhi. (Cardamom and its medicinal virtues.)

Ody, P. 1993. *The Herb Society's Complete Medicinal Herbal.* London: Dorling Kindersley. (Traditional use of cardamom.)

Pruthi, J. S. 1976. *Spices and Condiments.* New Delhi. 63. (Cultivation, production, harvest, storage, properties and uses of cardamom.)

Thorpes, 1945–1950. *Thorpe's Dictionary of Applied Chemistry.* London: Longmans, Green and Co. Vols. 1–10.

Yagna Narayan Aiyer, A. K. 1944. *Field Crops of India.* Bangalore: Government Press.

17

Asafoetida

Ferula asafoetida

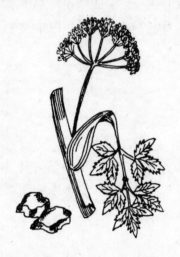

> Paste of hingu made with goat's urine cures the evil effects of grahas, insanity and fever.
>
> —Ayurveda Saukhyam of Todaraananda

Devil's Dung or God's Food?

Quite unaccustomed to its smell, and knowing hardly anything about its virtues, some European colonisers named this plant asafoetida ('the one that smells bad'). Some even went to the extent of calling it Devil's Dung. The Persians, on the other hand, glorified the plant by naming it God's Food.

Asafoetida in India

The name asafoetida is often attributed to the dried latex or oleogum oleoresin exuded by the living rhizome or rootstock or tap root of several species of *Ferula*. Although in certain parts of India, the entire plant is used as a fresh vegetable or in day-to-day dishes, asafoetida is more a medicine than a food. It is the major ingredient in many a digestive mixture (*Churan*) as it effectively expels the wind from the digestive tract.

Recent scientific studies have confirmed the medicinal usefulness of this plant.

The Profile

Botanical Name	:	*Ferula asafoetida* L.
English Names	:	Asafoetida, Devil's Dung, Food of the Gods.
Indian Names	:	Bengali, Gujarati, Hindi, Marathi, Punjabi & Urdu : *Hing*
		Kannada : *Hinger*
		Kashmiri : *Yang, Sap*
		Malayalam & Tamil : *Perungayam*
		Oriya : *Hengu*
		Sanskrit : *Agudagandha*
		Telugu : *Ingumo*
Family	:	Umbelliferae.
Appearance	:	A perennial herb with robust, carrot-shaped roots. Leaves, of two kinds: lower, simple, ovate and upper, much divided into numerous segments. Flowers in clusters, small, yellow.
Distribution	:	Grown in Punjab and Kashmir.
Medicinal Parts	:	Dried exudate from the living rootstock.

117

In Tradition

AILMENT	PRESCRIPTION
✤ Diabetes	: Mix 1/4 tsp asafoetida powder in 2 tsp bitter gourd juice. Take twice a day.
✤ Heart problems	: Eat 1/4 tsp asafoetida along with one large raisin every day.
✤ Gas problems	: Insert 1/4 tsp asafoetida into a ripe banana and eat.
✤ Gas, indigestion	: Roast slightly the following: 1 tbsp dried ginger, 1 tbsp each long pepper, cumin, curry leaves, ajwain and black pepper. Fry in 1 tsp gingelly oil 1 tsp asafoetida separately and mix all together and powder. Add a little rock salt. Store in a glass bottle. *Dosage:* Mix 1 tsp along with ghee and a little steamed rice.
✤ Stomach problems	: Dissolve 1 tsp asafoetida in 1 teacup hot water. Drench a cloth pad and foment the abdominal region.
✤ Stomach ache, liver problems	: Fry equal quantities of asafoetida, fenugreek, mustard seeds and turmeric powder in an adequate quantity of ghee. Grind into a fine powder. *Dosage*: 3 to 4 tsp along with 1 cup cooked rice.
✤ Kidney-pain	: Mix 1/4 tsp asafoetida in 2 tsp fresh ginger juice. Add a pinch of salt and sip.
✤ Earache	: Heat equal quantities of asafoetida,

garlic and calamus in a little neem oil. Strain and use as ear drops, when lukewarm.

❧ Headache : Grind 2 tsp tail pepper, 1 tsp each dried ginger, camphor and asafoetida either with an adequate quantity of rose water or milk into a smooth paste and apply.

❧ Toothache : Heat $1/2$ tsp asafoetida in 2 tsp lime juice. Soak a piece of cotton in this solution and place it in the tooth cavity.

❧ Sexual debility : Fry a small piece of asafoetida ($1/4$ tsp) in ghee. Add $1/2$ tsp banyan latex. Eat in the morning every day along with a banana.

❧ Asthmatic problems : Mix $1/4$ tsp asafoetida powder in 2 tsp honey and add $1/2$ tsp each betel leaf juice and white onion juice. Sip three times a day. (*Note:* Avoid yoghurt, buttermilk, banana, guava and fried food.)

Note: Individual results may vary.

In Science

Guenther, E. 1948–1952. *The Essential Oils*. 6 vols. New York: D. van Nostrand Co. Ltd. (Asafoetida's properties.)

Howes, F. N. 1949. *Vegetable Gums and Resins*. Mass: Waltham. The Chronica Botanica Co.

Kirtikar, K. R. and B. D. Basu. 1935. *Indian Medicinal Plants*. 4 vols. 2nd edn. Revised by E. Blatter et al. Allahabad: Lalit Mohan Basu. (Medicinal uses of asafoetida.)

Subrahmanyan, V. and M. Srinivasan. 1955. Asafoetida—Its origin, nature and place in human dietary and medicine. *The Bull. CFTRI (Mysore)* 5:27.

Wallis, T. E. 1946. *Text Book of Pharmacognosy*. London: J&A Churchill Ltd. (Medicinal uses of asafoetida.)

18

Fig

Ficus carica

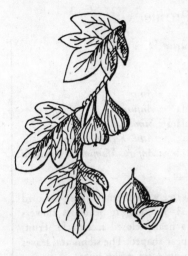

Figs are restorative, and the best food that can be taken by those who are brought low by long sickness...

—Pliny, *the Roman naturalist (A.D. 23/24–79)*

The Nutritive Coolant

The fig tree which traces its origin to the distant lands of the Mediterranean has enriched nutritional value in Indian households.

The nutritive index of fig, in comparison to others, shows its impressive value.

Fruit	Nutritive Index
Fig	11
Apple	9
Raisin	8
Date	6
Pear	6

The dried fruits are highly nutritive and contain iron, copper and other minerals including trace elements like zinc, Vitamins A and C and a high concentration, fifty to sixty per cent, of invert sugar.

Intake of fig cools down the body, stopping the effects of excessive heat such as nasal bleeding.

The Profile

Botanical Name	:	*Ficus carica* L.
English Name	:	Fig.
Indian Names	:	Hindi : *Anjir* Kannada : *Anjura* Malayalam : *Simayathi* Tamil : *Athi, Seemai Athi* Telugu : *Anjuru, Manjimedi, Simayatti*
Family	:	Moraceae.
Appearance	:	A small tree with alternate, long-petioled leaves. 3–5 lobed. It bears its flowers inside a nearly closed receptacle. Fruit, fleshy, pear-shaped. The stems and leaves contain an acrid milky juice.
Distribution	:	Cultivated in Uttar Pradesh, Rajasthan, Punjab, Andhra Pradesh and Maharashtra.
Medicinal Parts	:	Bark, leaves, leaf buds, roots, fruits (both fresh and dry), latex.

In Tradition

AILMENT	PRESCRIPTION
❧ Arthritic swellings	: Apply fresh latex (milk) of the tree on the affected areas.

❧ Deficiency : Soak 2 or 3 dried figs in 1 teacup
  in blood   water. Eat them along with milk next
                morning for a month.

❧ Diabetes : Eat 1 tsp seeds of the fig, separated
             from the pulp, along with 1 tsp honey
             every day for a few weeks.

❧ Inflammation : Eat 2 or 3 figs along with 1 teacup
  of spleen   curd twice a day for a few weeks.

❧ Constipation due : Take 2 or 3 figs after each meal.
  to diabetes

❧ Diarrhoea, : Mix 1 tsp powder of bark in 1 teacup
  stomach problems, buttermilk and drink daily for a few
  etc   days.

❧ Kidney-stones : Consume 1 teacup juice of fresh figs
                  frequently.

                : Boil 2 small fig pieces in 1 teacup water.
                  Take 2 to 3 times daily for a few weeks.

❧ Kidney-stones, : Boil 6 figs in 1 teacup water. Drink
  bladder stones   daily for a month.

❧ Eye problems : Boil 2 to 3 figs along with 1 tbsp
  due to *pitta*- raisins in 1 teacup milk. Drink every
  aggravation   morning during breakfast. (It is also a
                   brain tonic.)

❧ Halitosis, : Chew one or two tender leaves and
  mouth ulcer, etc leaf buds frequently and wash the
                    mouth with warm water.

123

❖ Loss of hair : Dry out 2 teacups fig roots in the shade for 3 days. Crush them and immerse in 1 teacup coconut oil for 15 days. Strain and bottle. Massage on scalp at bedtime. Leave on overnight.

❖ Mouth ulcer, sore throat, ulcer in uterus, etc : Mix 1 tsp powder of bark in 1 teacup milk. Add 1 tsp sugar to taste. Take daily for a few days.

❖ Excess menstruation in women : Grind 10 fresh leaf buds and apply on the lower abdomen below the navel for a few hours. Repeat this frequently.

❖ Leucorrhoea : Take equal quantities of the bark of the banyan and fig tree. Grind them into a fine powder. Mix 1 tbsp in 2 teacups water and use it as a vaginal douche.

❖ Boils, small tumours : Roast a fresh fig and cut into half. Make a poultice and apply.

❖ Early stages of leucoderma : Apply frequently the juice of leaves on the affected areas.

❖ Early stages of smallpox and chickenpox. : Include figs in your diet every day. (*Note:* Fig hastens the appearance of rashes.)

❖ Smallpox : Cut 2–3 figs into small pieces and cook in 1 teacup water. Cool. Add a pinch of saffron and eat twice daily.

❖ Warts : Apply the milky juice exuding from

the stems and leaves on the affected areas.

✤ Wounds : Mix 1 tbsp powder of bark in 1 teacup hot water and wash the wounds.

✤ Constipation, : Soak 2 or 3 dried figs overnight in
dry cough, 1 teacup water. Eat them along with
liver problems, 1 tbsp honey the next morning.
pitta-aggravation, Continue for a month.
physical weakness

Note: Individual results may vary.

In Science

Condit, I. J. 1947. *The Fig*. Mass: Waltham. Chronica Botanica Co. (A monograph.)

Corner, E. J. H. 1952. *Wayside Trees of Malaya*. 2 vols. Singapore: Government Printing Office.

Hayes, W. B. 1953. *Fruit Growing in India*. 2nd edn. Allahabad: Kitabistan. (Fig growing in India.)

Hill, A. F. 1952. *Economic Botany: A Text-book of Useful Plants and Plant Products*. 2nd edn. New York: McGraw Hill. (Fig and its importance in health and nutrition.)

Jamieson, G. S. 1943. *Vegetable Fats and Oils*. 2nd edn. New York: Reinhold Publication Corporation.

Kirtikar, K. R. and B. D. Basu. 1935. *Indian Medicinal Plants*. Revised by E. Blatter et al. Allahabad: Lalit Mohan Basu. (Fig and its medicinal value.)

Naik. K. C. 1949. *South Indian Fruits and their Culture*. Madras: P. Varadachary & Co. (Horticultural aspects of fig.)

125

HOME REMEDIES

Wehmer, C. 1935. *Die Pflanzenstoffe.* 2 vols. Jena: Gustav Fischer. 1929–31; Suppl. (In German)

Winton, A. L. and K. S Winton. *The Structure and Composition of Foods.* 4 vols. New York: John Wiley & Sons. (Chemistry and nutritional value of figs.)

Wren, R. C. 1950. *Potters Cyclopaedia of Botanical Drugs and Preparations.* 6th edn. Revised by R. W. Wren. London: Potter & Clarks Ltd. (Fig as a drug.)

19

Saunf

Foeniculum vulgare

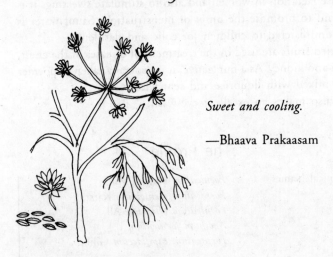

Sweet and cooling.

—Bhaava Prakaasam

Fennel cures Obesity

Pliny the Elder who lived in Rome in the 1st century A.D. discovered that fennel could cure obesity.

The Indian Fennel

India boasts of several varieties of fennel called saunf. The Indian varieties can be distinguished quite easily from their European cousins. Fennel fruits from Lucknow are priced very high as they are considered the best. They are used in several home remedies, particularly when there is feverishness, indigestion, vomiting.

Saunf Fruits

Saunf consists of the fruits of the fennel, often wrongly called seeds.

Saunf constitutes an excellent stomach and intestinal remedy. It is also a diuretic.

A hot infusion of the fruits is used in traditional medicine to increase lactation in women and also to stimulate sweating. It is also said to promote the onset of menstruation. Saunf water is also administered to children for colic and flatulence.

Dried fruits are used in the treatment of diseases of the chest, spleen and kidney. As a puragative, it is generally taken in powder form, mixed with liquorice and senna leaf.

It also makes an excellent eye-wash.

The Profile

Botanical Names	:	*Foeniculum vulgare* Mill. *Foeniculum foeniculum* Karst. *Foeniculum officinale* All. *Anethum foeniculum* L. *Foeniculum capillaceum* Gilib.
English Names	:	Fennel, Indian Sweet Fennel.
Indian Names	:	Bengali : *Mauri, Pan-Muhori.* Gujarati : *Variari, Wariyali.* Hindi : *Saunf, Bari Saunf* Kannada : *Badi Sopu* Marathi : *Badi-Shep* Tamil : *Sombu* Telugu : *Sopu, Pedda Jila-Kure*
Family	:	Umbelliferae.
Appearance	:	A tall, glabrous aromatic herb. Leaves, pinnately decompound. Flowers small,

yellow, in umbels. Fruit, ellipsoid, 6–7 mm in length, greenish or yellowish-brown.

Distribution	:	Cultivated as a winter crop in North India, Gujarat and Karnataka.
Medicinal Parts	:	Roots, fruits (often wrongly referred to as seeds).

In Tradition

AILMENT	PRESCRIPTION
❧ Joint pain	: Tie some saunf leaves in a cotton cloth. Warm them in a saucepan and apply on the affected parts when bearably hot.
❧ Anaemia	: Boil 6 tsp each crushed saunf and red rose petals in 1^1/$_2$ teacup water and strain. Take twice daily.
❧ Obesity, diabetes, indigestion, gas, constipation	: Roast saunf slightly on a heated ladle. Powder, sieve and bottle. Take ^{1}/$_2$ tsp of this *churan* twice a day along with warm water.
❧ Constipation	: Make a very fine powder of 1 tsp each of the following: saunf, dried ginger, senna leaves and rock salt. *Dose:* 1 tsp with water at bedtime.
❧ Diarrhoea	: Grind 3 tsp ginger along with 5 tsp saunf into a fine powder. Add enough honey to make a thick paste. *Dose:* 1 tsp in tea three times daily and before bedtime.

129

❧ Indigestion

: Grind 1 tsp each saunf, dried ginger and cloves into a fine powder. Add honey to make a thick paste. Preserve. Take 1 tsp after each meal and at bedtime.

: Make a fine powder of 1 tsp each saunf and cardamom. Dose: $1/4$ tsp with water twice daily after meals.

❧ Colic

: Boil 1 tbsp saunf in a glass of milk for 10 minutes. Strain and drink.

: Drink 1 teacup rose water, honey water or saunf water.

❧ Eye irritation, strain on eyes due to watching TV and excessive reading habits

: Boil $1/2$ tsp saunf in a cup of water till it is reduced to half. Cool. Use as eyedrops (*Caution*: Beware of contamination).

❧ Cough, hoarseness

: Gargle with warm saturated solution of saunf water.

❧ To stimulate lactation in nursing mothers

: Boil 2 tsp saunf in barley water and take twice or thrice a day.

❧ Breathing problems, cough, eye inflammation, fever, indigestion, phlegm formation, sneezing, stomach ache

: Boil 2 tbsp saunf in 1 teacup water till it is reduced to half. Filter. Take 1 tbsp every morning and evening for a few days. (This filtrate, when used to wash the eyes frequently, is reported to strengthen the eye muscles. It is a good cleansing lotion for inflamed eyes.)

❧ Cough : Add 1 to 3 drops saunf oil to 1 tbsp honey. Take a teaspoon at a time.

❧ Obesity : Boil well 2 tbsp saunf and 1 tsp chebulic myrobalan rind in 1 teacup water till the water is reduced to one-fourth of its original volume. Filter. Mix 1 tsp old honey and drink before breakfast on an empty stomach. *Note:* (1) This decoction should not be refrigerated or kept for the second day's use. (2) As we add chebulic myrobalan, no iron or aluminium vessel should be used. (3) This decoction can be boiled in a mud pot, enamel ware or in a silver utensil.

Note: Individual results may vary.

A Word of Caution

In excess, saunf stimulates menstruation in women. In very high doses, it can cause intoxication.

Saunf Tea, the Fat-Buster

Saunf tea extracts all of fennel's medicinal goodness, and can be substituted for tea and coffee.

Boil 1 tsp saunf in 1 cup toned milk for 5 to 10 minutes. Filter. Add sugar if necessary. Sip as hot as possible.

For those who suffer from obesity, saunf tea could be an ideal medicine.

In Science

Abyshev, D. Z. and I. A. Damirov. 1972. Coumarins and their production from fennel growing in Azerbaidzhan. *Azerb. Med. Zh.* 49:32; *Chem. Abstr.* 78:33848w. (Coumarins found in the roots of saunf.)

Hitokoto, H. et al. 1980. Inhibitory effect of spices on growth and toxin production of toxigenic fungi. *Appl. Environ. Microbiol.* *39*:818; *Chem. Abstr.* 1980, *93*:44284 V. (Powdered fennel inhibited the growth and toxin production of *Aspergillus* species.)

Kartha, A. R. S. and R. A. Khan. 1969. Proportions of 7–octadecenoic acids in seed-fats from ten umbelliferae species. London: *Chem. Ind.* 1869.

Kartnig, Th. et al. 1965. Some lipid containing materials from the roots and fruits of *Foeniculum vulgare*. *Fette Seifen Arstrichm.* *67*:10; *Chem. Abstr.* 1965. *63*:2048 g. (In German)

Kartnig, Th. 1965. Lipid substances contained in Umbelliferone fruits. *Pharm. Ztg.* 110:1051; *Chem. Abstr.* 64:7074a. (Long-chain acids isolated from saunf.)

Kostennikova, Z. P. et al. 1977. Evaluation of the quality of the Traskov anti-asthmatic mixture. *Farmtsiya* 25:60; *Chem. Abstr.* 1977, *86*:21820 h. (Saunf is an important ingredient in anti-asthmatic preparations.)

Kunzemann, J. and K. Herrmann. 1977. Isolation and identification of flavon(ol)-O-glycosides in caraway (*Carum carvi* L.), fennel (*Foeniculum vulgare* Mill.), anise (*Pimpinella anisum* L.) and coriander (*Coriandrum sativum* L.) and of flavone-C-glycosides in anise. I. Phenolics of species. *Z. Lebensm. Unters Forsch.* 164:194; *Chem. Abstr.* 87:166146y. (Isolation and identification.)

Lawrence, B. M. 1979. Progress in Essential Oils. *Perfumer Flavorist* 4:54. (An update of the extraction process.)

Nakaoki, T. et al. 1961. Medicinal Resources, XIX. Flavanoid of the leaves of *Nelumbo nucifera, Cosmos bipinnatus* and *Foeniculum vulgare*.

Yakugaku Zasshi 81:1158; *Chem. Abstr. 1962*, 56:1527 d. (Flavone-glycosides isolated from the aerial parts of fennel.)

Ohta, Y. and T. Miyazaki. 1959. Fenicularin, a quercetin-3-arabinoside from the leaves of *Foeniculum vulgare*. *Yakugaku Zasshi* 79:986; *Chem. Abstr.* 53: 20695a. (Flavóne-glycoside isolated from the aerial parts of fennel.)

Peyrone, L. et al. 1969. Existence of 1, 8-terpin in Chinese anise and sweet fennel oil (*Illicium verum* and *Foeniculum vulgare* var. dulce). *Bull. Soc. Chim. Fr.* 339. (The chemical constituent in fennel oil.)

Rao, B. S. et al. 1925. Notes on some Indian essential oils. *J. Indian Inst. Sci.* 8A:143;*Chem. Abstr.* 19: 3563–3565.

Rodriguez, M. M. et al. 1982. Determination of anethole in fennel (*Foeniculum vulgare* Mill.) *Acta Farm. Bonaerens* 1:75. (Anethole's presence was determined by spectroscopic methods.)

Sarkar, S. 1977. Occurrence of arachidic esters in *Foeniculum vulgare*. *Indian J. Chem.* 15B:583. (Long-chain esters isolated from the fruits of fennel.)

Scarpati, M. L. and O. Giovanna. 1957. Search for cynarin in plants containing other caffefyl derivatives. *Ann. Chim. (Rome).* 47:155; *Chem. Abstr.* 51:11495i. (Cynarin isolated from the aerial part of the fennel plant.)

Trenkle, K. 1972. Recent investigations on fennel (*Foeniculum vulgare.*) 2. The essential oil of fruits, herbs and root of the fruiting plants. *Pharmazie* 27:319.

20

Liquorice

Glycyrrhiza glabra

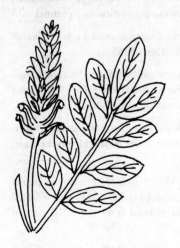

Chinese licorice (Glycyrrhiza uralensis): Roots and lower stems are used as a buffer in herbal prescriptions, act similar to adrenocortical hormones, and are effective against stomach ulcers and Addison's Disease.

—Xiao, Pei-Gen and Fu, Shan-Lin

Liquorice: A Bit of History

Liquorice has been known for thousands of years for its medicinal value.

It is one of the principal drugs mentioned by Susruta. It has been evaluated as *rasayana* by both Charaka and Susruta, in their respective treatises.

Vagabhatta however, prescribed it for the treatment of ulcer and jaundice. Its use is also referred to in *Granthi* and *Arbuda* in Ayurveda.

Its root has been in use in ancient Western herbalism as well. It was used as an expectorant, antitussive agent and as a sweetener.

For the Chinese, it is a drug for strengthening muscles and bones and for curing wounds. It is considered to be an aphrodisiac by them.

In India, the crude drug as well as its dried aqueous extract is mainly used in bronchial troubles.

Liquorice: A Bit of Chemistry and Pharmacology

Glycyrrhizin isolated from the root is the principal sweetening ingredient. On hydrolysis, it gives glycyrrhetic acid which possesses anti-inflammatory properties. Glycyrrhizin ointment is employed clinically for inflammatory skin diseases. Its anti-inflammatory activity is reported to be akin to that of cortisones.

Vagabhatta's prescription of liquorice for curing ulcer stands endorsed in several clinical trials made recently, notably by Revers, 1946 and Takagi and Ishii, 1967.

The Profile

Botanical Name	:	*Glycyrrhiza glabra* L.
English Names	:	Sweet Liquorice, Sweet-Wood, Liquorice Root.
Indian Names	:	Bengali : *Jashtimadhu*
		Hindi : *Mulethi, Mulahti*
		Kannada : *Yashtimadhukam*
		Malayalam : *Iratimadhuram*
		Sanskrit : *Madhuyasti*
		Tamil : *Atimadhuram*
		Telugu : *Yashtimadhukam*
Family	:	Fabaceae.
Appearance	:	Perennial plant found wild. The woody rootstock is wrinkled and brown on the

outside, yellow on the inside and tastes
sweet. The stem which is round on the
lower part and angular higher up bears
alternate, odd-pinnate leaves. Leaflets are
ovate and dark green in colour. Flowers,
yellow or purple or violet. Pods
compressed.

Distribution : Cultivated in Jammu and Kashmir,
Punjab and sub-Himalayan tracts. Large
quantities of roots are however imported.

Medicinal Parts : Rootstock.

Preparation and : Infusion/Decoction: 1 tsp rootstock in
Dosage 1 cup water. Take 1 cup a day.

In Tradition

AILMENT   PRESCRIPTION

❧ Jaundice : Make a fine powder of 1 tsp each
crushed liquorice root, chicory seeds
and rock salt. Take $1/2$ tsp with water
twice daily.

❧ Low B.P., fatigue : Add $3/4$ teacup crushed liquorice root
to 4 teacups cold water and allow it to
stand for 2 hrs. Then bring it quickly
to a boil and steep for 5 mts. Add this
to the bathwater in the tub.

❧ Peptic ulcer, : Take 1 cup infusion or decoction daily
kidney ailments for a month. (See The Profile for
preparation.)

❧ Peptic ulcer,   : Soak $1/2$ tsp liquorice root powder in
   muscular pain, etc   1 teacup water and leave overnight. Mix
   into the infusion 1 teacup rice gruel
   (cooked broken rice) and take every
   morning.

❧ Constipation   : Mix 1 tsp finely powdered liquorice
   root with 1 tsp jaggery. Add 1 cup
   water and drink.

❧ Aching eyes,   : Powder equal quantities of liquorice
   burning sensation   and cumin. Take $1/4$ tsp every day along
   during the   with 1 tsp honey for a month.
   discharge of urine,
   deterioration in
   vision, headache
   on one side

❧ Bad breath   : Cleanse the mouth with liquorice
   powder. After washing with water chew
   come saunf (1 tsp).

❧ Baldness   : Grind 2 tbsp each liquorice root and
   (not due to   seeds of dhatura (*Caution:* Poisonous)
   hereditary factors)   in milk cream along with $1/4$ tsp
   saffron. Heat this paste thoroughly in
   2 tbsp coconut oil, till charred. Apply
   on bald patches every night before
   going to bed, continuously. As dhatura
   is poisonous, keep this away from
   children and wash your hands after
   every application.

🌱 Baldness, dandruff, hair loss, etc

: Grind 1 tbsp root pieces in 1 teacup milk with 1/4 tsp saffron. Apply this paste on bald patches at bedtime continuously.

🌱 Myopia

: Mix 1/2 tsp liquorice root powder in equal quantities of ghee and honey. Take thrice daily along with milk before meals for a month.

🌱 Inflammation in mouth, mouth ulcers, etc

: Soak 1 tbsp crushed liquorice root in 2 teacups water for 2 to 3 hrs and use it for gargling frequently.

🌱 To remove yellowness in the eyes

: Very fine powder of liquorice is dusted into eyes (*Caution:* Proper care is to be exercised).

🌱 Sore throat

: Chew or suck a small piece of raw liquorice root.

🌱 Bronchitis

: Boil 2 tsp each crushed liquorice root and linseed in 2 teacups water for 10 mts. Strain and sweeten with 4 tbsp honey. Take 1 tsp twice or thrice a day.

🌱 Common cold

: Boil 1 tsp each liquorice and cinnamon with 1 tbsp ginger paste in 1 cup water for 10 mts. Filter. Add 1 tsp honey and drink.

🌱 Dry cough, sore throat, stomach upset, etc

: Boil 1 tsp liquorice root in 1 teacup water and strain. Mix in 1 tsp honey and take daily for a few days.

❧ Corns : Mix 1 tbsp liquorice powder with
$1/2$ teacup mustard oil and make a
smooth paste. Rub it into the hardened
skin at bedtime.

❧ Soothing : Apply 1 tsp finely powdered root on
effect on skin the skin.

❧ Wounds : Mix 1 tbsp liquorice root powder with
equal quantities of ghee and honey.
Apply it as ointment over wounds.

❧ Anorexia, emacia- : Use 1 tsp rootstock with 1 cup water
tion, chronic joint to make an infusion or decoction. Take
problems, etc 1 cup a day.
(It also allays thirst)

❧ Ache, burning : Slightly roast 5 tbsp each liquorice, rind
sensation in the of chebulic myrobalan and cardamom.
anal region, Grind them into a fine powder. Take
bleeding $1/4$ tsp of this mixture twice a day along
with 1 teacup water and 1 tsp honey.

Note: Individual results may vary.

The Science

Chopra, R. N. and S. L. Nayar. 1956. *Glossary of Indian Medicinal Plants.* New Delhi: Council of Scientific and Industrial Research. (Liquorice, the drug.)

Balbaa, S. I. et al. 1975. A phytochemical study of *Glycyrrhiza glabra* Linn. growing in Egypt. *Bull. Fac. Pharma. Cairo Univ.* 14(1):213–229; *Chem Abstr.* 87:206410. (Chemistry of liquorice.)

Finney, R. S. H. and A. L. Tarnocky. 1960. The Pharmacological properties of glycyrrhetic acid hydrogensuccinate (disodium salt). *J. Pharm. Pharmacol.* 12:49. (A pharmacological study.)

Gujral, M. L. et al. 1959. Antiarthritic activity of *Glycyrrhiza glabra L. Indian J. Physiol Pharmacol.* 3:39. (The use of liquorice in treating arthritis.)

Gujral, M. L. et al. 1961. Anti-arthritic activity of Glycyrrhizin in adrenal-ectomised rats. *Indian J. Exp. Bio.* 6:232. (Role of glycyrrhizin as an anti-arthritic agent.)

Ikram, M. and K. A. Zirvi. 1976. Chemistry and pharmacology of liquorice (genus *Glycyrrhiza*). *Herba Pol.* 22 :312–320. (Chemical and pharmacological evaluation of liquorice.)

Rai, A. N. et al. 1980. Effect of *Yashtimadhu* (*Glycyrrhiza glabra* Linn) on conjunctivitis. *J. Res. Ayur. Sid.* 1,1:21–24. (Clinical parameters and microbiological studies confirmed the drug's efficacy particularly in acute conditions. Cortisone-like anti-inflammatory potential is also reported.)

Revers, F. E. 1946. Has liquorice juice (*succue liquirides*) a healing action on gastric ulcer? *Med. Tjdschr. Gencesk.* 90:135. (In the treatment of gastric ulcer.)

Takagi, K. and Y. Ishii. 1967. Peptic ulcer inhibiting properties of a new fraction from licorice root (FM100). 1. Experimental Peptic Ulcer and general pharmacology. *Arzneimittel-Forsch 17:*11544. (In the treatment of peptic ulcer.)

Zaini, F. et al. 1993. Inhibition of mutagenicity in *Salmonella typhimurium* by *Glycyrrhiza glabra* extract, etc. *Planta Medica 59*(6) 502–50.

21

Chinese Hibiscus

Hibiscus rosa-sinensis

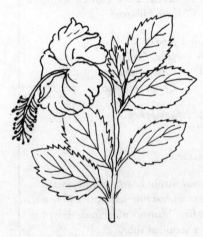

Dried flower powder enhances masculinity and soothes burning sensation during urination.

—Dr. Thirumalai Natarajan

Shoe-Flower

Chinese Hibiscus is also known as Shoe-Flower. It is cultivated as an ornamental plant in gardens.

Science endorses Tradition

Its flowers are astringent, hypoglycaemic and considered to have an aphrodisiac quality. They are extensively used in treating alopaecia, burning sensation in the body, diabetes, menstrual disorders, piles, fever, cough, menorrhagia and ulcer.

Recent scientific findings have confirmed their antifertility properties. Their definitive action in the treatment of arterial hypertension stands upheld by clinical studies.

The Profile

Botanical Name	:	*Hibiscus rosa-sinensis* L.
English Names	:	Rose of China, Shoe-Flower, Chinese Rose, Chinese Hibiscus.
Indian Names	:	Bengali : *Jaba*
		Hindi : *Jaba, Gurhar*
		Tamil : *Chappaathu, Chemparaththai*
Other Vernacular Names	:	*Jasum, Japapushpam.*
Family	:	Malvaceae.
Appearance	:	Glabrous shrub. Leaves simple alternate. Flowers of varying colours, often red. Petals five. Stamens numerous, united to form a staminal tube.
Distribution	:	Grown in gardens all over the country.
Medicinal Parts	:	Flowers, flower buds, petals, stamens, roots.

In Tradition

AILMENT	PRESCRIPTION
❧ Heart problems	: Boil 2 petals of hibiscus in 1 teacup water and strain. Mix in a teaspoonful honey and take once a day for a few days.

142

❧ Weak heart : Boil 5 flowers in 1 teacup water till the volume is reduced to $1/2$ teacup. Add 1 tsp sugar and 1 teacup cow's milk. Take once a day.

❧ Cystitis, irritable conditions of the urinogenital tract, urinary diseases : Boil 5 flowers in 2 teacups water. Mash and filter. Add 1 tsp sugar candy. Take 1 tsp of this decoction once or twice a day for a few days.

❧ Burning sensation while passing urine, sexual debility : Dry some flower buds under the sun. Powder them. Take 1 to 2 tsp with honey or ghee once or twice a day. This powder can also be added to a glass of milk and taken after the milk is boiled.

❧ Urinary disorders : Soak 10 flowers in a jug of water overnight and use this frequently for drinking.

❧ Hair loss, dullness of hair : Heat 10 flowers in 2 teacups coconut oil till charred. Filter and use as hair oil.

❧ Sexual debility : Cut the stamens from 5 flowers and boil in a cup of milk and drink every day at bed time.

Note: Individual results may vary.

A Word of Caution

During the course of treatment, patients are advised to avoid meat.

In Science

Agarwal, S. K. and R. P. Rastogi. 1971. Triterpenoids of *Hibiscus rosa-sinensis* Linn. *Indian J. Pharm.* 33:41–42. (A chemical investigation.)

Agarwal, S. L. and S. Shinde. 1967. Studies on *Hibiscus rosa-sinensis*, Part II. Preliminary pharmacological investigations. *Indian J. Med. Res.* 55:1007. (Hibiscus can bring down high BP.)

Batta, S. K. and G. Santhakumari. 1971. The antifertility effect of *Ocimum sanctum* and *Hibiscus rosa-sinensis*. *Indian J. Med. Res.* 59:777. (Role of hibiscus in population control.)

Bhakuni, D. S. et al. 1969. Screening of Indian plants for biological activity, Part II. *Indian J. Exptl. Biol.* 7:250. (Antispasmodic action of hibiscus.)

Bhatnagar, S. S. et al. 1961. Biological activity of Indian plants. Part I. Antibacterial, antitubercular and antiviral action. *Indian J. Med. Res.* 49:799. (Anti-fungal and anti-bacterial action of hibiscus.)

Chopra, R. N. et al. 1956. *Glossary of Indian Medicinal Plants.* 133. New Delhi: Council of Scientific and Industrial Research. (Laxative and demulcent action of hibiscus.)

Dwivedi, R. N. 1977. Role of *Japapushpa (Hibiscus rosa-sinensis)* in the treatment of arterial hypertension. A trial study. *Jour. Res. Ind. Med. Yoga & Homeop.* 12(4): 31–36.

Gupta, M. L. et al. 1971. A study of antifertility effect of some indigenous drugs. *J. Res. Indian Med.* 6(2):112.

Kholkute, S. D. et al. 1976. Screening of indigenous medicinal plants for antifertility potentiality. *Planta Med.* 29:151. (Flower extract of hibiscus shows anti-estrogenic action.)

Kholkute, S. D. and K. N. Udupa. 1974. Antifertility activity of *Hibiscus rosa-sinensis*. *J. Res. Indian Med.* 9(4):99. (Flower extract administered from day 1 to day 10 of pregnancy in rats was found to be the most effective in preventing pregnancy.)

Kholkute, S. D. et al. 1976. Effect of *Hibiscus rosa-sinensis* Linn. on estrus cycle and reproductive organs in rats. *Indian J. Exptl. Biol.*

14:703. (The extract played a role in reducing weight of ovary and uterus, pituitary and uterine atrophic changes in experimental animals.)

Kurup, P. N. V. et al. 1979. *Handbook of Medicinal Plants*. New Delhi.

Nadkarni, A. K. 1954. *Indian Materia Medica*. Bombay. (A wealth of data on medical plants.)

Prakash, A. O. 1980. Effect of *Hibiscus rosa-sinensis* Linn. extracts on *corpus lutea* of cyclic guinea-pigs. *Sci.& Cult.* 46:330. (Evidence of anti-estrogenic action of hibiscus.)

Sethi, N. et al. 1986. Teratological study of an indigenous antifertility medicine, *Hibiscus rosa-sinensis* in rats. *Arogya Jour. Health Sci. 12*:86–88. (A study of monstrosities and abnormal formations.)

Singh, M. P. et al. 1982. Antifertility activity of a benzene extract of *Hibiscus rosa-sinensis* flowers on female albino rats. *Planta Med. 44*(3):171–174.

Singh, M. S. and S. B. Lal. 1980. Cytostatic and cytotoxic effects of flower extract of *Hibiscus rosa-sinensis* on spermatogenically and andogenically active testes of a non-scrotal bat, *Rhinopoma kinneari* Wroughton. *Indian J. Exptl. Biol. 18:1405.* (Flower extract depleted germ-cells and sperms.)

Singh, N. et al. 1978. A pharmacological investigation of some indigenous drugs of plant origin for evaluation of their antipyretic, analgesic and anti-inflammatory activities. *J. Res. Indian Med. Yoga and Homeo.* 13(2):58. (A valuable evaluation of hibiscus.)

Singh, R. and R. Singh. 1972. Screening of some plant extracts for anti-viral properties. *Technology* (Sindri) 9:415. (Antiviral properties of hibiscus.)

Singh, S. P. 1977. A pharmacological evaluation of antipyretic, analgesic and anti-inflammatory activities of some indigenous drugs. *Indian J. Pharm.* 9(1):80.

Singh, S. P. et al. 1978. Antifertility studies of some indigenous plants. *Indian J. Pharmacol.* 10(1):88. (Hibiscus proves useful in controlling human fertility.)

HOME REMEDIES

Tiwari, P. V. 1974. Preliminary clinical trial on flowers of *Hibiscus rosa-sinensis* as an oral contraceptive agent. *J. Res. Indian Med.* 9(4):96.

Wahi, S. P. et al. 1974. Pharmacognostical studies on *Hibiscus rosa-sinensis* L. *Jour. Res. Ind. Med.* 9(4):84–95.

22

Mango

Mangifera indica

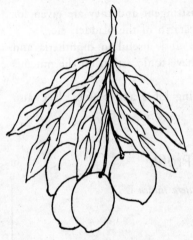

The year in which I don't eat enough mangoes should be deleted from my life-span.

—Rabindranath Tagore

King of Indian Fruits

The mango, often referred to as the king of fruits, is considered very auspicious by the Hindus. Its fruits, wood, leaves, etc have found their way into many religious ceremonies.

There are hundreds of varieties of mangoes grown in India. The mango which has a thin rind, a small stone and bristleless pulp is considered the best. The North Indian varieties Dasheri and Langda fall under this category.

The ideal way to eat mangoes is to cool them by keeping them immersed in cold water. Then they should be sucked or chewed. Plain water should not be taken with mangoes. More often, it is recommended to drink milk along with mangoes. The mango-milk combination is reported to reduce the acidity of the mango. It is also considered an ideal food—the milk supplements protein which is lacking in the mango.

Mangoes cleanse the body by eliminating toxins. The emergence of boils on the body after eating a lot of mangoes is an indicator of the cleansing action of mangoes.

In case mangoes are eaten in excess, the best antidote is to eat a few jamuns. Drinking an infusion of cumin may also quicken its digestion.

Dried mango flowers are astringent and they are given for diarrhoea, chronic dysentery, catarrh of the bladder, etc.

The bark is astringent too. It is useful in diphtheria and rheumatism. It is believed to have tonic action on the mucous membrane.

The gum is used in dressing kibes and scabies. It is also considered anti-syphylitic.

The Profile

Botanical Name	:	*Mangifera indica* L.
English Name	:	Mango.
Indian Names	:	Gujarati : *Amri*
		Hindi : *Aam*
		Kannada : *Mavu*
		Marathi : *Amba*
		Malayalam : *Amram, Mavu*
		Sanskrit : *Amra, Chuta*
		Tamil : *Mangai*
		Telugu : *Mamidi, Mavi*
Family	:	Anacardiaceae.
Appearance	:	Huge tree with a big, thick stem and dark brown bark. Leaves long, wavy, glabrous. Fruits juicy. Seed hard, often referred to as stone.

148

Distribution	:	Grown extensively in Uttar Pradesh, Punjab, Maharashtra, Andhra Pradesh, West Bengal and Tamil Nadu.
Medicinal Parts	:	Bark, leaves, leaf buds, flowers, fruit (raw), kernel, root.

In Tradition

AILMENT	PRESCRIPTION
❧ Rickets	: Mix 1 tsp powder of dried raw mangoes with 1 tsp honey. Take twice.
❧ Toothache, gum inflammation	: Boil 2 tbsp mango flowers and tender buds in 2 teacups water and wash the mouth frequently.
❧ Diabetes	: Take 1 tsp crushed tender leaf buds of mango and neem.
	: Grind 1 tbsp each dried mango flowers, dried tender mango buds and dried seeds of jamun into a very fine powder and store. *Dose*: 1 tsp along with hot water every morning for 40 days.
❧ Spleen enlargement	: Add 1 tsp honey to a teacup of ripe mango pulp. Take thrice a day.
❧ Diarrhoea	: Take 1 tbsp dried powdered mango kernel and roast it with an equal quantity of powdered aniseed. Sieve it. Take 1 tsp of this mixture along with some warm water.

	: Apply 1 tbsp paste made of the inner portion of mango bark around the navel.
❧ Diarrhoea, dysentery	: Take 1 tsp dried mango flowers, mixed with 1 tsp honey.
❧ Digestive and liver troubles	: Suck a ripe mango and top it with a glass of milk.
❧ Intestinal worms	: Slice and dry the kernel. Mix 1 tbsp fenugreek and powder. Take 1 tsp in buttermilk.
❧ Dysentery	: Grind 1 tsp each mango flowers, tender mango buds and pomegranate flowers into a fine paste. Mix into a teacup of buttermilk and drink.
❧ Bleeding piles, intestinal worms	: Mix 1/2 tsp powder of the kernel in 1 teacup whey and drink.
❧ Fever	: Grind a few roots of the mango tree into a fine paste and apply on the palms and soles of the patients.
❧ Baldness	: Rub on the scalp 1 tbsp oil in which raw mangoes have been preserved for over one year. Repeat this treatment frequently.
❧ Earache	: Extract 1 tsp juice from mango leaves. Slightly warm and use as ear drops when bearably hot.

❧ Nose bleeds : Extract a few drops of the juice of the soft kernel and instil in nostrils.

❧ Pain in the eyes : Grind a raw mango to pulp in a blender and heat it gently to make a poultice.

❧ Teeth problems : Burn a handful of dry leaves. Add 1 tsp each mustard oil and common salt to the ash. Use as toothpowder.

❧ Burns caused by fire : Burn a handful of mango leaves to ashes and apply this on the affected parts.

❧ Cracked feet : Mix 1 tsp mango tree gum with 1 tbsp water and apply on the sole.

❧ Eczema : Mix 2 tbsp each of the bark powder of babul Acacia and mango. Boil in 5 teacups water. Allow the vapour to foment affected parts. After fomentation, anoint with ghee.

❧ Wounds : Boil 2 tbsp powder of bark in 1 teacup water. Strain through a muslin cloth and wash the wound.

❧ Body weakness : Sprinkle the following on a platter of mango slices: 1 tsp honey, a pinch of saffron, cardamom and rose water. Take twice daily.

❧ Heat exhaustion, heat stroke : Cook an unripe fruit in hot ashes. Extract the pulp and mix with water and 1 tbsp sugar, and take.

❧ Prickly heat   : Boil 2 raw mangoes in 2 teacups water. Cool. Squeeze out the pulp. Add salt or sugar or both to taste. Drink at least once a day.

Note: Individual results may vary.

A Word of Caution

People who suffer from psoriasis, skin diseases and stomach ulcer are advised to avoid mangoes.

In Science

Burkill, I. H. 1935. *A Dictionary of Economic Plants of Malay Peninsula.* 2 vols. London: Crown Agents for the Colonies. (On the uses of Malayan mangoes.)

Chandler, W. H. 1950. *Evergreen Orchards.* Philadelphia: Lea & Fabiger. (How to grow mangoes.)

Dastur, J. F. 1951. *Useful Plants of India and Pakistan.* Bombay: D. B. Taraporevala & Sons.

Department of Agriculture, Hyderabad. 1954. *The Mango: A Souvenir.*

Kirtikar, K. R. and B. D. Basu. *Indian Medicinal Plants.* Revised by E. Blatter et al. Allahabad: Lalit Mohan Basu.

Mayer, F. 1943. *The Chemistry of Natural Colouring Matters.* Translated and revised by A. H. Cook. New York: Reinhold Publication Corporation. (Pigments in the mango.)

Naik, K. C. 1958. *Horticulture in South India.* New Delhi: Ministry of Food and Agriculture. (Cultivation of mangoes.)

Naik, K. C. and S. R. Gangolly. 1950. *A Monograph on Classification and Nomenclature of South Indian Mangoes.* Madras: Superintendent of Government Press.

Singh, L. B. 1960. *The Mango: Botany, Cultivation and Utilization.* London: Leonard Hill (Books) Ltd. (An introduction.)

Singh, L. B. and J. L. Bose. 1961. Chemical examination of mango panicles (*Mangifera indica* L). *J. Sci. Indust. Res.* 20B:296. (Chemistry of panicles.)

Winton, A. L. and K. B. Winton. 1935. *The Structure and Composition of Foods.* 4 vols. New York: John Wiley.

23

Pudina

Mentha arvensis

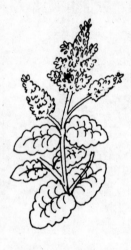

Pudina fights germs and parasites.

—Priyanighantu Shatpushpadivarga

Pudina and the Three Great Mints

Fieldmint is a common herb in the Indian kitchen, popularly known as pudina.

It is one of the Three Great Mints. The other two mints are peppermint and spearmint.

All these mints have a soothing action on the nerves and digestion.

Fieldmint contains large amounts of the element of ether, whose action is soothing, clarifying and expanding. Through its ethereal nature, it helps relieve mental and emotional tension. It also clears the mind, senses and blood of impurities.

The whole plant, leaves, stems and their extracts exhibit antispasmodic, carminative, stomachic, refrigerant, stimulant emmenagogue, diuretic, antifertility, anti-ovulatory, anti-bacterial and anti-fungal properties in laboratory and clinical experiments.

There is no better way to consume fieldmint than as a tangy pudina chutney, an irresistible appetiser in Indian cuisine. (See: Pudina Chutney, page 158.)

The Profile

Botanical Name	:	*Mentha arvensis* L.
English Name	:	Fieldmint.
Indian Names	:	Bengali, Gujarati, Hindi, Marathi,
		Punjabi & Urdu : *Pudina*
		Kashmiri : *Pudiyanu*
		Malayalam : *Muthina*
		Tamil & Telugu : *Podina*
Family	:	Labiatae.
Appearance	:	A spreading aromatic herb with dark green, crinkled, scented leaves. Flowers, small, lilac, in small bunches.
Distribution	:	Mainly grown in the Western Himalayas, Kashmir, Punjab, Kumaon and Garhwal.
Medicinal Parts	:	Leaf, stem, whole plant, extracts.

In Tradition

AILMENT	PRESCRIPTION
❧ Abdominal gripe, indigestion	: Chew 1/4 tsp seeds of mint and drink a glass of warm water.

❧ Abdominal pains, fever, heart burn, hiccups, jaundice, poor digestion, painful urination, stomach ache

: Add 1 tbsp leaves to 1 teacup water. Take twice or thrice a day.

❧ Colic

: Boil 1 tsp leaves in 1 teacup water for 3 mts. Drink twice a day.

❧ Biliousness, dyspepsia, indigestion, jaundice, morning sickness, piles, nausea

: Mix 1 tsp each fresh juice of mint and lime along with 1 tbsp honey. Take 3 times a day.

❧ Indigestion, insomnia, nausea, nervousness, loss of sensitivity in taste buds

: Steep 1 tbsp leaves in 1 teacup water for 30 mts. Drink the infusion. (*Note:* Do not boil.)

❧ Indigestion

: Mix 1–3 drops of mint oil with 5 teacups water and drink whenever needed.

❧ Nausea

: Boil 1 tsp mint leaves along with $1/2$ tsp small cardamom in a glass of water and drink.

❧ Nausea

: Boil 1 tsp dried mint leaves with a small bit of ginger, $1/2$ tsp black pepper and 1 tbsp palmyrah sugar in 1 teacup water and drink.

❧ Fever

: Clean, crush and boil a handful of mint leaves along with a paste made of

156

$^1/_2$ tsp black pepper, $^1/_2$ tsp long pepper and 1 tsp dry ginger powder in 2 teacups water, till reduced to 1 teacup. Filter and divide into 3 equal doses and take 3 times a day.

❧ Bad odour, infection in mouth
: Powder the dried plants. Use as toothpowder.

❧ Headache
: Apply 1 tsp fresh leaf juice on forehead.

❧ Infection in ears and nose
: Extract 1 tbsp leaf juice. Soak cotton-wool and squeeze a few drops into ears or nose.

❧ Teeth problems
: Grind a handful of the dried leaves into a very fine powder. Add 1 tbsp salt ' and use it as toothpowder.

❧ Delayed menstruation
: Powder 1 tsp dried leaves and take with 1 tsp honey, thrice daily.

❧ Burning sensation in legs
: Tie a handful of leaves along with 5 tbsp salt in a cloth. Warm it in a saucepan. Apply on the foot when bearably hot.

❧ Urticaria
: Boil 1 tsp mint with 2 tsp raw sugar in a glass of water and drink.

Note: Individual results may vary.

Pudina Chutney

Ingredients:
2 tbsp fresh coriander leaves, chopped
1 tbsp fresh pudina leaves, chopped
1 clove garlic, crushed
1 green chilli, finely chopped or ground
1 tbsp fresh lemon juice
1 tbsp thick coconut milk or yoghurt. Salt to taste.

Put all the ingredients into a blender and run on high for a few seconds to mix well. Add more yoghurt or coconut milk as desired to make the consistency you prefer.

You can use this as bread-spread or eat it with chapati or cooked rice.

In Science

Aswal, B. S. et al. 1984. Screening of Indian plants for biological activity. Part XI. *Indian J. Exptl. Biol.* 22:487. (Pudina shows diuretic properties.)

Bodhankar, S. L. et al. 1971. Effect of *Mentha arvensis* Linn on fertility in female albino rats. *Bull. P.G.I. Chandigarh* 5(2):66. (Extract of the plant exhibits anti-implantation effects.)

Bodhankar, S. L. et al. 1973. Mechanism of action of indigenous infertility agents. *Bull. P.G.I. Chandigarh* 7(3):127. (Studies on anti-implantation effects indicate that the alcoholic extract might have anti-zygotic effect.)

Chaudhury, R. R. and M. Haq. 1980. Review of plants screened for antifertility activity. *Bull. Medico-Ethno-Bot. Res.* 1(3):408–419. (Alcoholic extract of leaves in dosages of 125–250 mg/kg p.o. on rats exhibited antifertility effect; in 500 mg/kg p.o., it produced hundred per cent anti-implantation effect.)

Chaurasia, S. C. et al. 1976. Activity of some volatile oils against

Phytophtora parasitica var. *Piperina. Indian Drugs* 13:9. (The essential oil of pudina was found to possess highly significant anti-fungal property against *Phytophtora parasitica* and *Curvularia lanata.*)

Chaurasia, S. C. and A. Kher. 1978. Activity of essential oil of three medicinal plants against various pathogenic and non-pathogenic fungi. *Indian J. Hosp. Pharm.* 15:139. (Highly significant anti-fungal properties of pudina confirmed.)

Chomchalow, N. and N. Pichitakul. 1977. Studies on mint in Thailand. *Proceedings of the Third Asian Symposium on Medicinal Plants and Spices.* Colombo: Unesco. (Menthol is the major component of pharmaceuticals such as balm, cough-drops, inhalants and medicine for the treatment of stomach disorders.)

Chopra, R. N. et al. 1956. *Glossary of Indian Medicinal Plants* 165. New Delhi: CSIR. (Pudina, which is a stimulant and emmenogogue, also possessed diuretic properties.)

Garg, S. K. et al. 1978. Screening of Indian plants for antifertility activity. *Indian J. Exptl. Biol.* 16(10):1077–1079. (Extract of pudina leaves produced 60% inhibition of pregnancy.)

Kapoor, M. et al. 1964. Antiovulatory activity of 5 indigenous plants in rabbits. *Indian J. Med. Res.* 62:1225. (Anti-ovulatory properties of pudina confirmed.)

Kholkute, S. D. et al. 1976. Screening of indigenous medicinal plants for antifertility potentiality. *Planta Med.* 29:151.

Palevitch, D. 1978. *Mentha*: an important medicinal and aromatic plant. *Agrotike* 1975 (1):9–11. (In Greek)

Ramesh Chandra. et al. 1978. A clinical trail of Gasex in gastro-intestinal symptoms. *Probe* 27(4):330–333. (2 tablets of Gasex, containing pudina, thrice daily was found effective in flatulence and abdominal discomfort, acidity and nausea.)

Sampurna, T. and S. S. Nigam. 1980. Efficacy of Indian essential oils in combination against *Salmonella typhii. Indian Drugs Pharmaceut. Ind.* 15(b):7. (Pudina's essential oil in combination with other oils obtained from other *Mentha* species and eucalyptus showed highly active anti-bacterial effect.)

Sanyal, A. and K. C. Varma. 1969. *In vitro* antibacterial and antifungal activity of *Mentha arvensis* var. *piperascens* oil obtained from different sources (Letter to editor). *Indian J. Microbiol.* 9(1):23. (The oil was found effective against *Aspergillus niger* and *Curvularia lunata.*)

Singh, S. P. 1977. *Search for effective antifertility agents from indigenous plant sources.* Thesis for M.D. Pharmacology. K.G. Med. Coll. Lucknow. (Antifertility efficacy of pudina confirmed.)

Singh, S. P. et al. 1978. Antifertility studies of some indigenous plants. *Indian J. Pharmacol.* 10:88.

Singh, S. P. 1982. Brief resumé of the antifertility studies conducted by P. R. U., Lucknow. *Symposium on Family Welfare Research Programme sponsored by CCRAS, Ministry of Health and Family Welfare, New Delhi.* May 1982. (Pudina's antifertility role documented.)

24

Bitter Gourd

Momordica charantia

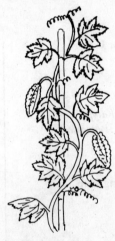

Karvellaka kills germs.

—Bhava Prakasha

The Diabetic's Plant

Bitter gourd is a highly sought-after plant by traditional physicians who prescribe it for diabetic patients.

The significant hypoglycaemic activity of the fruits of *Momordica charantia* has been tested by many scientists. Several clinical trials have also proved that oral administration of the fruits causes a decrease in blood sugar level. Water extract of the fruit was experimentally found to be more effective than powder of dry fruits. Smaller varieties of bitter gourd are preferred for diabetes.

Charantin, an alkaloid from the fruits, has been identified to be as potent a hypoglycaemic agent as tolbutamide.

The drug improves digestion, calms down the sexual urge,

cures anaemia, anorexia, leprosy, ulcers, jaundice, flatulence and piles.

Bhisagarya records that there are three varieties of bitter gourd. However, the Kerala physicians recognize only 2 types: paval (*Momordica charantia*) and kaattupaval (*Momordica tuberosa*). The latter is a rather rare wild species with tuberous roots.

In Profile

Botanical Name	:	*Momordica charantia* L.
English Name	:	Bitter Gourd.
Indian Names	:	Hindi : *Karela*
		Malayalam : *Pavel, Kaippa*
		Tamil : *Parkai, Paavakkai*
Family	:	Cucurbitaceae.
Appearance	:	A climbing or trailing herb.
Distribution	:	All over India.
Medicinal Parts	:	Fruits, leaves, seeds.

In Tradition

AILMENT	PRESCRIPTION
✤ Enlargement of spleen	: Take 1 tbsp bitter gourd fruit juice every day for a few days.
	: 4 tbsp juice of green bitter gourd taken for 1 week to 10 days.
✤ Diabetes	: Mix 1 tbsp each amla fruit juice and

bitter gourd fruit juice, and take once every morning for two months.

: Take equal quantities of fruits of amla, Java Plum and bitter gourd. Extract their juice. 1 tbsp twice daily.

: Extract 2 tsp juice from bitter gourd leaves. Mix in 2–3 pinches of ground asafoetida. Take daily in the morning.

✤ Intestinal worms, sugar problems

: Take 5–10 seeds and crush them. Fry them in a little ghee. Take twice daily.

✤ Bleeding piles, intestinal worms

: Take 1 tbsp juice extracted from bitter gourd leaves. Mix into a glassful of buttermilk and take every morning.

✤ Haematuria (Blood in urine)

: Vegetable dish made from one green banana, two drumsticks and one bitter gourd to be included on a regular basis in the diet.

✤ Piles

: Mix 2 tbsp root powder with a little water into a fine paste and apply on the affected parts.

✤ To increase milk flow in lactating mothers

: Grind a handful of leaves into a fine paste and apply on breasts.

✤ Leucoderma

: Frequent intake of bitter gourd juice (1 to 2 tbsp everyday). (*Note*: Salt-free diet is recommended. Exposure to heat is to be avoided.)

❦ Burning sensation in feet and palms

: Grind a handful of bitter gourd leaves into a smooth paste and apply on the affected areas of feet and palms frequently.

❦ Leprous wounds, skin eruptions

: Dry a handful of leaves and make them into fine powder. Dust on the affected areas.

❦ Measles

: Extract 1 tbsp juice from bitter gourd leaves. Mix in 1 tsp honey and 2 pinches turmeric powder (or ground turmeric paste). Take twice a day.

❦ Wounds

: Take 1 tbsp juice of a ripe bitter gourd fruit and mix in 1 tsp sugar. Apply on affected parts.

Note: Individual results may vary.

A Word of Caution

Excess intake of bitter gourd leaves can cause diarrhoea and vomiting. To stop such side effects restrict food to a diet of 1 tbsp ghee and 1 teacup cooked rice.

People with skin ailments are advised to avoid the intake of bitter gourd and brinjal.

In Science

Akhtar, M. S. et al. 1981. Effect of *Momordica charantia* on blood sugar level of normal and alloxan diabetic rabbits. *Planta Med.* 42(3):205–212. (Bitter gourd's use in treating diabetes.)

Central Council for Research in Ayurveda & Siddha. 1990. *Pharmacological Investigations of Certain Medical Plants and Compound Formulations used in Ayurveda and Siddha.* New Delhi. (A very useful reference volume.)

Day, C. et al. 1991. Hypoglycaemic effect of *Momordica charantia* extracts. *Planta Med.* 56(5):428–429.

Dutta, P. K. et al. 1981. Studies on Indian medicinal plants. Part 64: Vicine, a favism-inducing toxin from *Momordica charantia* Linn. seeds. *Indian J. Chem.* 20B:669. (Vicine, the toxin.)

Handa, G. et al. 1991. Hypoglycaemic principles of *Momordica charantia* seeds. *Indian J. Nat. Prod.* 6(1):16–19.

Higashino, H. et al. 1992. Hypoglycaemic effects of Siamese *Momordica charantia* and *Phyllanthus urinaria* extracts in streptozotocin-induced diabetic rats (The 1st report). *Nippon Yakurigaku Zasshi* 100(5):415–21. (English Abstract)

Jamwal, K. S. and K. K. Anand. 1962. Preliminary screening of some reputed abortificient indigenous plants *(Karela). Indian J. Pharm.* 24(9):218–220.

Kar, A. et al. 1970. Anoretic, psycho-pharmacological and cardio-vascular actions of the essential oil of *Momordica charantia. East Pharma* 13 (147):43–46. (The oil found to be non-toxic.)

Karunanayake, E. H. et al. 1984. Oral hypoglycaemic activities of some medicinal plants of Sri Lanka. *J. Ethnopharmacol.* 11(2):223–231. (A Sri Lankan report confirming the hypoglycaemic activity of bitter gourd.)

Kedap, P. and C. H. Chakrobarti. 1982. Effects of bitter gourd (*Momordica charantia*) seeds and glibendamide in streptozotocin induced *Diabetes mellitus. Indian J. Exp. Biol.* 20(3):232–233. (Efficacy of bitter gourd seeds.)

Khan, R. A. & Onkar Singh. 1992. Anti-diabetic profile of *Momordica charantia. Hamdard Medic.* 35(1):76–79. (Anti-diabetic profile of bitter gourd.)

Kierti, S. et al. 1982. Effect of *Momordica charantia* (*Karela*) extract on blood and urine sugar in *Diabetes mellitus*—Study from a diabetic clinic. *Clinician* 46(1):26–29.

Kurup, P. A. 1956. Studies on plant antibiotics—Screening of some Indian medicinal plants. *J. Sci. Indust Res.* 15C(6):153–154. (Antibiotic role of bitter gourd.)

Lotlikar, M. M. and M. R. R. Rao. 1966. Pharmacology of hypoglycaemic principle isolated from the fruits of *Momordica charantia. Indian J. Pharm.* 28(5):129–133. (The alkaloid, charantin lowers blood glucose by 42%.)

Meir, P. and Z. Yanis. 1985. An *in-vitro* study on the effect of *Momordica charantia* on glucone uptake and glucose metabolism in rats. *Planta Med.* 1:12–16. (Reconfirmation.)

Nahar, N. 1993. *Medicinal Plants in the Treatment of Diabetes, in Traditional Medicine.* New Delhi: Oxford-IBH. 205–209. (Pulp-juice of *Momordica charantia* had significant fasting blood glucose lowering effect in rats.)

Pabrai, D. N. and K. B. Sehra. 1962. Effect of *Momordica charantia* on blood sugar in rabbits. *Indian J. Pharm.* 24(2): 48. (Hypoglycaemic effects observed.)

Pabrai, D. N. and K. B. Sehra. 1962. Effect of *Momordica charantia* on blood sugar in rabbits. *Indian J. Pharm.*24(9):209–213.

Padmini, K. and C. H. Chakrabarti. 1982. Effects of bitter gourd (*Momordica charantia*) seed and glibenclamide in streptozotocin induced *Diabetic mellitus. Indian J. Exptl. Biol.* 20(3):232–235. (Seed found to be hypoglycaemic.)

Prakash, A. O. and R. Mathur. 1976. Screening of Indian plants for antifertility activity. *Indian J. Exptl. Biol.* 14(5):623–626. (Abortifacient role of bitter gourd.)

Sharma, V. N. et al. 1960. Some observations on hypoglycaemic activity of *Momordica charantia. Indian J. Med. Res.* 48(4):471–477. (Fruit juice 12 cc/kg. shows hypoglycaemic effect on rabbits.)

Srivastava, Y. et al. 1993. Anti-diabetic and adaptogenic properties of *Momordica charantia* extract. An experimental and clinical evaluation. *Phytotherapy Res.* 7(4):285–289. (More recent studies on the efficacy of bitter gourd in fighting diabetes and stress.)

Tennekoon, K. H. et al. 1994. Effect of *Momordica charantia* on key hepatic enzymes. *J. Ethnopharmacol.* 44(2):93–97. (An enzyme study.)

Upadhyaya, G. L. and M. C. Pant. 1986. Effects of water and other extracts of bitter gourd powder on blood sugar and serum-cholesterol level in albino rabbits. *Jour. Diabet. Assoc. India* 26(1):17–19.

Verma, J. P. and J. S. Aggarwal. 1956. A note on component fatty acids of the oil from the seeds of *Momordica charantia* Linn. *J. Indian Chem. Soc.* 33:357. (Chemistry of the seed oil.)

Vimla Devi, M. et al. 1977. Hypoglycaemic activity of leaves of *Momordica charantia. Indian J. Pharma.* 39(6):167. (Leaves of bitter gourd show hypoglycaemic activity comparable to that of tolbutamide.)

Zafar, R. and Neerja. 1991. *Momordica charantia*—A Review. *Hamdard Medic.* 34(3) 49–61.

25

Curry Leaf

Murraya koenigii

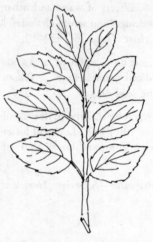

Curry leaf, the germ-killer.

—Guna Paadham

Sought-After Tree of the Commons

The curry leaf tree is the most common tree in India, abundantly growing in the deciduous forests and jungles of the country.

It is the most sought-after aromatic in South Indian cuisine, flavouring *dal, sambar, rasam, kari,* etc.

There is a marked difference between the tender and the mature leaves of this plant.

Tender leaves have less protein, less fat, less sugar, less starch, less mineral content, less crude fibre as compared to mature ones. However, they contain volatile oil and oleo-resins in abundance. Hence for flavouring purposes, tender leaves are preferred.

The leaves, in general, strengthen the body, increase appetite, eliminate body heat and fever. They impart brightness to the eyes and guarantee blackness of hair.

The juice of the root is taken to relieve pain associated with the kidneys.

The Profile

Botanical Names	:	*Murraya koenigii* L. *Bergeria koenigii* L.	
English Name	:	Curry Leaf.	
Indian Names	:	Assamese	: *Narsingha, Bisharhari*
		Bengali	: *Barsanga, Kariaphulli*
		Gujarati	: *Goranimb, Kadhilimbdo*
		Hindi	: *Karipatta, Meetha Neem, Kathneem*
		Kannada Malayalam,	: *Karibevu*
		Tamil	: *Kariveppilei*
		Marathi	: *Karhinimb, Poospala, Gandla, Jhirang*
		Oriya	: *Barsan, Basango, Bhursunga*
		Punjabi	: *Curry-Patia*
		Telugu	: *Karepaku*
Family	:	Rutaceae.	
Appearance	:	A large shrub or a small tree.	
Distribution	:	Widely cultivated in Tamil Nadu, Maharashtra and North India for its leaves which are used for flavouring curries. Also grows widely in Indian forests.	
Medicinal Parts	:	Bark, root, leaves, fruits and fruit pulp.	
Preparation	:	Paste of fresh leaves, powder of dried leaves, juice of roots or leaves, infusion or decoction of leaves.	

In Tradition

AILMENT	PRESCRIPTION
✤ Diabetes due to hereditary factors, obesity	: Eat 10 fresh, fully grown curry leaves every morning for 3 to 4 months. (Avoid fatty foods, sweets and alcohol.)
✤ Bilious vomiting	: Mix 1 tsp finely powdered tree bark in 2 teacups cold water and take 2 or 3 times.
	: Mix 1 tsp finely ground bark in cold water and drink.
✤ Constipation	: Mix 1 tsp dried curry leaf powder with 1 tsp honey and eat twice or thrice a day.
✤ Constipation, indigestion	: Dry a handful of leaves in the shade. Add 1 tsp each pepper, cumin and dried ginger. Add salt to taste. Powder all of them together. Mix this powder in ghee and eat with steamed rice.
✤ Diarrhoea, dysentery, piles	: Mix juice of 15–20 tender leaves with 1 tsp honey and drink.
✤ Dysentery	: Eat 5 to 10 raw, tender leaves.
✤ Nausea	: An infusion of 1 tbsp roasted leaf soaked in 1 teacup water.
✤ Nausea, *pitta*-aggravation, stomach upset	: Make a chutney of a handful of fresh leaves by adding 1 tsp tamarind, one fried red chilli and salt to taste. Eat with rice or chapatis.

❧ Nausea, vomiting : Soak a handful of curry leaves in 4 cups of hot water for 2 hours. Take $1/2$ teacup of the filtrate three times a day.

❧ Loss of taste sensitivity in the tongue, stomach discomfort : Put a handful of crushed leaves, bark and root of curry leaf tree in drinking water.

❧ Stomach trouble : Extract juice from 15 to 20 curry leaves and mix it with buttermilk. Take twice or thrice daily.

❧ Vomiting : Roast 15–20 leaves and make an infusion by mixing 1 teacup water into it. Drink.

❧ To strengthen the stomach and improve digestive functions. : Mix 1 tbsp juice of curry leaves in a glassful of buttermilk and drink daily, twice or thrice.

❧ To relieve kidney pain : Mix 1 tsp juice of the roots with 1 tsp honey and take.

❧ Early development of cataract : Fresh curry leaf juice suffused in the eyes. (*Caution*: handle with care to avoid infection.)

❧ Falling hair, dandruff (it helps in blackening the hair and imparts lustre) : Mix equal quantities of dried curry leaves, lime peel, shikakai, fenugreek seeds and green gram and grind them finely. Store and use as a substitute for soap or shampoo.

ᴪ Premature   : Take juice or chutney made of curry
  greying of hair   leaves everyday.

                : Boil a handful of curry leaves in 1 tbsp
                 coconut oil till charred. When cool,
                 use as hair tonic to retain natural
                 pigmentation.

ᴪ Morning sickness : Mix juice of 15–20 tender curry leaves
                 with 2 tsp lime juice and 1 tsp sugar.
                 Take in the morning.

ᴪ Burns   : Apply curry leaves as poultices over
                 affected areas.

ᴪ Insect bites   : Mix the fruit pulp with an equal
                 quantity of lime juice and apply on
                 affected parts.

Note: Individual results may vary.

In Science

Anwar, F. et al. 1972. Terpenoid alkaloids from *Murraya koenigii* Spreng.
VII—Synthesis of 4-0-methylmahanine and related carbazoles.
Experientia 28:769. (Synthesis of chemical ingredients found in
curry leaves.)

Anwar, F. et al. 1973. Synthesis of murraycine: Oxidation with DDQ
of the activated aromatic methyl group of the alkaloids of *Murraya
koenigii* Spreng. *Indian J. Chem.* 11:1314–1315. (On murraycine,
an alkaloid found in curry leaves.)

Gowda, P. H. R. et al. 1990. Uses and cultivation of curry leaf. *Lal
Baugh* 31(1):49–50. (The horticultural aspects of curry leaves.)

Khan, B. A. et al. 1995. Hypoglycemic action of *Murraya koenigii* (Curry Leaf) and *Brassica juncea* (Mustard): Mechanism of Action. *Indian J. Biochem. Biophys.* 32 (2):106.

Khan, B. A. et al. 1995. Haematological and histological studies after curry leaf (*Murraya koenigii*) and mustard (*Brassica Juncea*) feeding in rats. *Indian J. Med. Res.* 102:184.

Kureel, S. P. et al. 1969. Terpenoid alkaloids from *Murraya koenigii* Spreng.: II—The constitution of cyclomahanimbine, bicyclomahanimbine and mahanimbidine. *Tetrahedron Lett.* 44:3857–3862. (A study of the alkaloids in curry leaves.)

Kureel, S. P. et al. 1969. New alkaloids from *Murraya koenigii* Spreng. *Experientia* 25:790.

Kureel, S. P. et al. 1970. Two novel alkaloids from *Murraya koenigii* Spreng. mahanimbicine and bicyclomahanimbicine. *Chem.& Ind.* 950.

Kureel, S. P. et al. 1970. Terpenoid alkaloids from *Murraya koenigii* Spreng. IV. Structure and synthesis of mahanimbinine. *Experientia* 26:1055.

Prakash, V. and Natarajan. C. P. 1974. Studies on curry leaf (*Murraya Koenigii L*). *Proc. Symposium: Development and Prospects of Spice Industry in India.* Mysore: Assn. Food Scientists and Technologists. p. 65. (A scientific study.)

Santhosh Kumari, K. S. and K. S. Devi. 1990. Hypoglycaemic effect of a few medicinal plants. *Ancient Sc. of Life* 9(4):221–223.

26

Banana

Musa paradisiaca

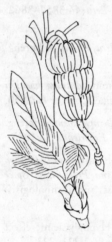

The banana promotes fertility and brings prosperity when used to decorate marriage halls.

—The Puranas

Harbinger of Prosperity

The Hindus believe that Lakshmi, the goddess of wealth resides on a banana leaf. Traditionally bananas have always been associated with prosperity and happiness.

Indians have not ignored this belief, and the Indian republic is, statistically speaking, the second largest producer of bananas in the world.

One-fourth of what is produced in India comes from a single state: Tamil Nadu. This state alone cultivates around 80 varieties of banana. Among them, Malai, Mondan, Poovan, Peyan and Rastali are the most well-known varieties with yellow fruits. Other varieties are: Green Nendran, Robusta, Karpooravalli, Dwarf Cavendish, etc.

While Poovan is considered highly useful for patients suffering from constipation and piles, Peyan helps patients suffering from smallpox and ulcer. However, people with *vata*-complaints should avoid this variety.

Malai increases blood production. It is easily digestible and a very good remedy for constipation. It cools down the body and controls *pitta*-aggravation.

Rastali is much sought after by connoisseurs. It is considered the king of bananas and hence is the most expensive. Although its taste and flavour are excellent, it has little or no medicinal use.

The edible rootstock of banana has several curative properties too. Venereal diseases, psoriasis, skin-infections, blood-infections, deficiencies in the blood—all these are reported to be cured by this insignificant part of the tree.

The fibres of the sheath of the stem are used in weaving a special type of fabric, worn by elderly people and priests.

The juice of banana flowers is said to cure diarrhoea, bleeding piles, burning sensations in hands and feet, cough, blood in stools, leucorrhoea, intestinal worms, psychological disorders due to *pitta*-aggravation, anal pain and menorrhagia.

The unripe fruits are reported to possess several medicinal properties. They are used in the treatment of *pitta*-aggravation, bleeding piles, nausea, stomach disorders, cough, excess urination, excess salivation, ulceritis, collitis, etc. They are also effective in increasing red blood corpuscles. However, in excess, they induce gas in stomach.

Unlike the unripe fruits, ripe fruits are mildly laxative in nature. They cool down the body. They could be red, green, yellow or mottled; small, medium or big. They are the real body-builders for growing children as they are loaded with calcium, potassium, sodium, phosphorous, sulphur, magnesium, iron and vitamins.

Traditionally there is a belief that by eating food on a banana leaf platter (as in traditional South Indian households), one wards off infections and food-poisoning. In addition, the following benefits accrue: improvement of eye-sight and retention of black-pigment and melanin in the hair (in other words, postponement of greying).

The Profile

Botanical Names	:	*Musa paradisiaca* L. *Musa sapientum* L.
English Names	:	Banana, Plantain, Kadali.
Indian Names	:	Hindi : *Kela* Kannada : *Baelehannu* Malayalam : *Kadalivaala, Kshetrakadal* Sanskrit : *Kadali* Tamil : *Kadali Vaalai* Telugu : *Kadalamu, Ariti*
Family	:	Musaceae.
Appearance	:	A tall herb with aerial pseudo stem, dying after flowering. Leaves, large, oblong, narrowed to base. Flowers in spikes, drooping with conspicuous bracts, dull-brown. Fruits berries in several clusters, generally golden yellow on ripening.
Distribution	:	Native of India and Malaya. Extensively cultivated throughout India, particularly in Assam, Madhya Pradesh, Bihar, Uttar Pradesh, Andhra Pradesh, Maharashtra, Kerala, Karnataka and Tamil Nadu.
Medicinal Parts	:	Root, stem, sheath, leaf, flower, fruit.

In Tradition

AILMENT	PRESCRIPTION
✦ Anaemia, deficiencies in blood, urinary diseases	: Mix 1 tbsp juice of amla with a ripe, mashed Nendran banana and eat twice or thrice a day.
✦ Kidney-stones	: Include the inner white portion of banana stem at least thrice a week in the diet. (Radish could be an alternative.)
✦ Acidity, anaemia, diabetes, intestinal worms, leprosy	: Burn some of the roots in the fire. Collect the ash. Take $1/4$ teaspoonful of this ash mixed with honey for a few days.
✦ Constipation, body weakness, heart weakness, intestinal ulcers	: Regular intake of ripe bananas.
✦ Diarrhoea	: Mash 1 ripe banana along with a pinch of salt and 1 tsp tamarind pulp. Take twice a day.
	: Mix 2 tbsp flower juice with $1/2$ cup curd and take once or twice a day.
✦ Indigestion	: Take a ripe banana along with a cup of milk as a night-cap.
✦ Piles	: Boil a mashed ripe banana in 1 teacup milk and take twice or thrice a day.

❧ Cough
: Mix 1/4 tsp black pepper powder with a mashed ripe Nendran banana and eat twice or thrice a day.

❧ Leucorrhoea, stomach disorders
: Mix 2 tbsp flower juice with 2 tsp powdered palmyrah candy.

❧ TB
: Mash a ripe banana along with 1/2 cup curd, 1 tsp honey and 1 teacup coconut water and take twice a day.

❧ Bed sores, burns on the body, smallpox
: Apply honey on the length and breadth of a banana leaf and lie on it for a few hours. Ensure its contact with the affected parts.

❧ Boils, psoriasis, skin-irritation
: Tie a fresh thin banana leaf on the affected area.

❧ Burns
: Mash a ripe banana and apply on burns. Bandage with betel leaves.

❧ Burns
: Crush the flowers or leaves and extract the juice. Apply on affected areas.

❧ Burns caused due to fire, hot water, hot oil, etc
: Take the thin buds of banana leaves. Bandage directly on affected areas. Tie the upper part for two days and then lower parts for two more days.

❧ Burning sensation on inner side of the feet, and eyes
: Mash 1 ripe banana along with a little curd and water; take twice a day.

✤ Skin-afflictions, wounds	: Dip a muslin cloth in coconut oil and spread on the affected area. Over this tie up a thin banana leaf like a bandage.
✤ Jaundice, smallpox, typhoid	: Mash a ripe banana along with 1 tbsp honey and eat twice a day for a few days.
✤ Anaemia, *pitta*-aggravation, polio, TB, throat-blockage	: Take a ripe Nendran banana along with 1 tbsp honey.
✤ Body weakness	: Cook 1 cup shredded flowers and add it to the meal.

Note: Individual results may vary.

A Word of Caution

Ripe banana fruits in excess can cause dysentery.

Banana flowers, in excess, may result in fluid-retention in body tissues.

Home-Made Moisturizer

Here is an easy way to make your own dry skin moisturizer.

Mash one ripe banana thoroughly. Mix in an equal quantity of warm olive oil. Blend them together into a fine spreadable paste.

Use as face pack.

In Science

Banerji, N. et al. 1982. A new 9, 19-cyclotriterpene from flowers of *Musa paradisiaca* (banana). *Indian J. Chem.* 21B: 387. (The chemical in banana flowers.)

Banerji, N. and A. K. Das. 1984. Isolation of a new 9, 19-cyclotriterpene from flowers of *Musa paradisiaca* (Banana). *J. Instn. Chem. India* 56:147.

Chattopadhyay, S. et al. 1967. Activation of peritoneal microphages by sitoindocid IV, an antiulcerogenic acylsterylglycoside from *Musa paradisiaca*. *Planta Med.* 53(1):16–18. (Bananas used in ulcer patients.)

Chopra, R. N. et al. *Glossary of Indian Medicinal Plants*. And its *Supplement* 72, 1969. New Delhi: CSIR. (Bananas drive away intestinal worms and is of significant use in otalgia, colitis, hypertension, nephritis, gout, etc.)

Dhar, M. L. et al. Screening of Indian Plants for biological activity, Part IV. *Indian J. Exptl. Biol.* 11:43, 1973. (Banana's anti-carcinogenic properties.)

Dharnidharka, V. R. et al. 1994. Use of banana-leaves in Stevens-Johnson syndrome (Letter). *Paediatr. Dermatol.* 11(3):280–281.

Dutta, P. K. et al. 1983. A tetracyclic triterpenoid from *Musa paradisiaca*. *Phytochemistry.* 22:2563.

Goel, R. K. et al. 1985. Effect of biological variables on the antiulcerogenic effect of vegetable plantain (bananas). *Planta Med.* No. 2:85–88. (Bananas as a cure for ulcer.)

Gomathy, R. et al. 1990. Hypoglycaemic action of pectin present in the juice of the inflorescence stalk of plantain. (*Musa sapientum*)—Mechanism of action. *J. Biosc.* 15(4): 297–303. (At a dose of 20 mg/100 gm body-weight, pectin shows significant hypoglycaemic effect in rats.)

Jain, S. R. and S. N. Sharma. 1967. Hypoglycaemic drugs of indigenous origin. *Planta Med.* 15:416. (Flower extract of banana reduced blood sugar levels in normal rabbits.)

Jain, S. R. 1968. Hypoglycaemic principle in *Musa sapientum* and its isolation. *Planta Med.* 16:43.

Osim, E. E. and J. O. Ibu. 1990. The effect of plantain (*Musa paradisiaca*) on DOCA-induced hypertension in rats. *Intl. J. Pharmacog.* 29(1):9–13.

Rao, V. V. et al. 1994. Hypoglycaemic effect of *Musa sapientum*. *Filoterapia* 65(1):65–67.

Roy, S. N. and S. Mukherji. 1979. Influence of tannins on certain aspects of iron metabolism. Part I. Absorption and excretion in normal anaemic rats. *Indian J. Biochem. Biophys. 16:93.* (Green bananas can cure anaemia.)

Roy, S. N. and S. Mukherji. 1979. Influence of food tannins on certain aspects of iron metabolism. Part II . Storage and transport in normal and anaemic rats. *Indian J. Biochem. Biophys.* 16:99. (Green banana tannin was found to contain high concentration of radioactive iron. Serum iron concentration increased with administration of banana.)

Roy, S. N. and S. Mukherji. 1979. Influence of food tannin on certain aspects of iron metabolism. Part III. *Indian J. Biochem. Biophys.* 16:151. (Tannin from green bananas might aid in iron utilization in anaemia.)

Sairam, T. V. 1987. Healing power of bananas. (Letter to the editor) *The Hindu* Oct. 18.

Sanyal, A. K. et al. 1961. Banana and gastric ulcer. (Letters to the editor) *J. Pharm. Pharmacol.* 13:318. (Bananas in the treatment of gastric ulcers.)

Sanyal, A. K. et al. 1963. Banana and experiment peptic ulcer (Letters to the editor) *J. Pharmacol.* 15:283. (Bananas in the treatment of peptic ulcers.)

Sanyal, A. K. et al. 1963. Banana and restraint ulcer in albino rats. (Letters to the editor.) *J. Pharmacol.* 775. (Anti-ulcer activity of bananas.)

Sanyal, A. K. et al. 1965. Studies on peptic ulceration. Part I: Role of banana in phenylbutazone-induced ulcers. *Arch. Int. Pharmacodyn. Ther.* 149–393.

Sanyal, A. K. et al. 1965. Studies on peptic ulceration, Part II. Role of banana inrestraint and prednisolone-induced ulcers in albino rats. *Arch. Int. Pharmacodyn. Ther.* 155:244.

Sinha, S. N. et al. 1961. Some obervations on 5-hydroxytryptamine content of edible fruits and vegetables and its effect on gastric activities. *Indian J. Med. Res.* 49:691. (Banana extract useful against chronic ulceration and perforation, caused by repeated histamine injection.)

Wadood, A. et al. 1990. Effect of *Musa sapientum* on blood glucose levels of normal and alloxan-treated diabetic rabbits. *Pakistan J. Med. Res.* 28(3):169–175.

27

Nutmeg

Myristica fragrans

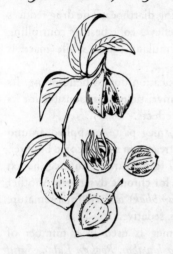

Nutmeg imparts tejas, strength and flavour.

—Guna Paadham

Fruit, Nut and Aril

Mace and nutmeg are two distinctly different spices produced from a single fruit. While nutmeg is the dried kernel, mace is the dried reticulated aril. When the peach-like nutmeg fruit bursts open, mace is seen as an attractive bright scarlet cage closely enveloping the hard, black, shining seed. The mace is removed gently, flattened, dried and is called the typical 'blade of mace'. On drying its original scarlet colour turns reddish brown and becomes brittle. Both were in use in India as a spice and as a medicine as early as 700 BC. They are generally known as baking spices as they are ideal flavouring agents in doughnuts.

The drug was known to the Greeks, Romans and Arabs long before it was known to the Europeans in the Middle Ages.

The Intoxicant Spice

Nutmeg is aromatic and bitter. It tends to be sweeter and more delicate than mace.

It is a household name in treating diarrhoea. The drug reduces the motility of the intestine and relieves colic besides controlling diarrhoea. It is considered a stimulant tonic, while mace is considered aphrodisiac.

Nutmeg is known for its intoxication due to benumbing. Its volatile constituents, particularly myristicin, is responsible for its pharmacological as well as toxic effects.

In some rural households, nutmeg paste is applied around the eyes. It is believed that by this treatment eyes become brighter.

In Ayurveda, *Jatiphaladi Bhati* (a mixture of nutmeg, borax, mica, dhatura and opium) is used for chronic dysentery. Another preparation (*Jatiphaladi Bhati Stambhak*) is used for premature ejaculation. *Jatiphaladi Churna* is sedative.

In the Unani tradition, nutmeg is used in a number of preparations: *Itrifal Ghudadi, Hab Jawahar, Roghan Kalan, Sufuf Longa, Majun Izragi, Majun Nankhwa Muski,* etc. In the last two preparations, mace is used while in the rest nutmeg is one of the ingredients.

The Profile

Botanical Name	:	*Myristica fragrans* Houtt.
English Name	:	Nutmeg.
Indian Names	:	Bengali, Gujarati, Hindi, Marathi,

Punjabi and Urdu	:	*Jaiphal, Jaivitri*
Kannada	:	*Jayikai, Japatre*
Kashmiri	:	*Zaaphal, Jaabvatur*
Malayalam		
and Tamil	:	*Jaadhikka,*
		Jaadhipatri
Oriya	:	*Jaiphala*
Sanskrit	:	*Jatiphala*
Telugu	:	*Jajikai, Japatri*

Family	:	Myristicaceae.
Appearance	:	Small evergreen tree with smooth greyish-brown bark. Leaves alternate, smooth and dark-green. Flowers small, creamy yellow, inconspicuous and unisexual. Fruit is peach-like. Fruit cover is hard, encasing a soft brown seed smelling like varnish. This is the nutmeg of commerce. A fleshy irregular covering which covers the hard seed coat is the mace.
Distribution	:	Grown on a small scale in Nilgiris, Kerala, Assam, Karnataka, West Bengal, etc.
Medicinal Parts	:	Kernel, aril, oil.

In Tradition

AILMENT	PRESCRIPTION
❧ Depression, hiccups, indigestion, insomnia, irritability, morning sickness	: Mix 1/8 tsp nutmeg powder with 1 tbsp freshly extracted amla juice. Take 3 times a day.

❧ Colic pain : Nutmeg, sweet flag and chebulic myrobalan—all the 3 are rubbed on a grinding stone. The paste obtained is used as a carminative and anti-spasmodic medicine. (*Dose:* $1/8$ tsp.)

❧ Colic pain, diarrohea : Take $1/8$ tsp finely ground nutmeg along with 1 tsp jaggery and 1 tsp ghee. (*Note:* A little dried ginger can also be added to take care of the irritant toxins.)

❧ Dehydration due to diarrhoea, particularly in cholera : Soak half a nutmeg in 2 teacups water for over 2–3 hours. Take 1 tsp of this infusion and mix in 1 teacup fresh coconut water. Drink twice or thrice a day.

❧ Diarrhoea : Add $1/8$ tsp nutmeg powder and 1 tsp ginger paste to $1/2$ teacup yoghurt diluted with $1/2$ teacup water and drink.

❧ Diarrhoea, caused by indigestion of food : Insert $1/8$ tsp nutmeg powder inside a ripe banana and eat.

❧ Dysentery : Add $1/8$ tsp powdered nutmeg to hot milk and take. (*Caution:* Do not prolong this treatment.)

❧ Gas problems : Finely powder the following: nutmeg 2 tsp, $1/4$ tsp dried ginger; mix and store. Take $1/8$ tsp along with a little warm water before meals. (*Caution:* Do not prolong this treatment.)

❧ Cough,
headache
(on one side),
stomach ache

: Mix 1 tsp each of the following powders and store: camphor, nutmeg, cardamom and cloves. Take 2 pinches with warm water.

❧ Halitosis or
bad breath

: Chew a small bit of mace as it is or wrapped in betel leaves (*Caution*: It is habit-forming with serious side-effects).

❧ Headache

: Make a paste of nutmeg and a grain of opium in cow's milk and apply to the forehead.

❧ Running nose

: Rub a nutmeg and a grain of opium on a smooth grinding stone along with some cow's milk. Apply this paste on forehead and nose.

❧ Toothache

: Apply nutmeg oil on affected parts.

❧ Deficiency
in semen

: Rub mace and nutmeg on a grinding stone with some milk. Fry a mixture of 1 tsp each finely ground long pepper, cloves, seeds of drumstick, khuskhus, seeds of peepul. Add the milk and heat. Take 1 tsp (*Caution*: Do not prolong this treatment).

❧ Sexual debility

: Mix $1/8$ tsp nutmeg powder in 1 tsp honey and take with a half-boiled egg an hour before going to bed.

❧ Eczema, ringworm

: Rub a nutmeg against a smooth stone slab with a little water and make a paste. Apply on affected parts. (*Note*:

It is believed by some rural, old-fashioned practitioners that instead of water, one's own early morning saliva can be used for better results.)

❧ Pimples : Grind equal quantities of nutmeg, black pepper and sandalwood and apply frequently.

❧ Body-pain, : Boil 3 tbsp powdered nutmeg in
breathing pro- 1 teacup sesame oil. Cool and apply
blems, neuralgia, on affected parts.
rheumatic pain,
sciatica

❧ Sleeplessness : Rub a nutmeg lightly against a smooth
and irritability in grinding stone in milk and feed
children children who cry out at night without
any apparent reasons. (*Caution:* It may
cause addiction on prolongation. Dosage
should be one pinch.)

Note: Individual results may vary.

A Word of Caution

Nutmegs should not be taken frequently. They should be taken in very small doses: not more than $1/8$ tsp. In excess, they excite the motor cortex and produce convulsions. They cause lesions in the liver and have a narcotic effect.

Even a teaspoon of nutmeg can produce toxic symptoms: giddiness with hallucination, burning in the stomach, nausea, vomiting, restlessness, etc.

In addition to hallucinations and elation, eating nutmegs can produce stomach-pain, double-vision, delirium and other symptoms of poisoning.

Eating as few as two nutmegs can cause death.

In Science

Forrest, J. E. and R. K. Heacock. 1972. Nutmeg and Mace. The psychotropic spices from *Myristica fragrans*. *Lloydia* 35:440.

Gopalakrishnan, M. et al. 1979. Identification of the mace pigment. *J. Food. Sci. Technol.* 16:261. (Lycopene has been identified as the colouring matter.)

Kalbhen, D. A. 1971. Nutmeg as a Narcotic: A contribution to the chemistry and pharmacology of nutmeg (*Myristica fragrans*) *Angew. Chem. Inter. Ed.* 10:370. (Misuse of nutmeg, which was introduced in Europe as an abortifacient, caused poisoning.)

Khandeparker, U. K. and R. D. Kulkarni. 1981. Anti-fatigue effect of indigenous drug 'geriforte' in rats. *Indian Drugs* 18:346. (Nutmeg as a constitutent contributed to anti-fatigue property of the drug.)

Lal, S. D. and L. Kamlesh. 1980. Plants used by the Bhat community for regulating fertility. *Econ. Bot.* 34:237. (The Bhat community has been using nutmeg preparations as an abortifacient).

Novotelnova, N. P. et al. 1964. Sclerol from wastes from manufacture of nutmeg oil. USSR, 161, 842 April 1; *Chem. Abstr.* 1964, 61:4145. (Sclerol was isolated as a by-product of nutmeg distillation.)

Pathak, S. P. and V. N. Ojha. 1957. Components and glycosides of nutmeg butter. *J. Sci. Fd. Agric.* 8:537.

Purushothaman, K. K. and A. Sarda. 1980. Chemical examination of the aril of *Myristica fragrams*. *Bull Medico-Ethnobot. Res.* 1:223.

Sethi, S. C. and J. S. Agarwal. 1952. Stabilization of Edible Fats by Spices and Condiments. Part I. *J. Sci. Industr. Res.* 11B:46. (Nutmeg fruit effectively check the development of rancidity in vegetable oils.)

Sherry, C. J. et al. 1979. Effect of the terpene fraction of nutmeg on the behaviour of young chicks. *Planta Med.* 36 :49. (The low boiling essential oil fractions of nutmeg induced increase in total average duration of sleep in chicks.)

28

Black Cumin

Nigella sativa

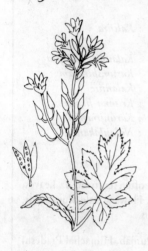

Black cumin cures fevers.

—Bha Pra Haritakyadivarga

Pest Repellent and Contraceptive

Black cumin is the dried seed-like fruit of a small herb originally from the Mediteranean region. It is cultivated in Assam, Bengal, Bihar, Himachal Pradesh and Punjab.

It is useful in mild puerperal fever and in skin-eruptions. It is also used for scorpion-stings in the villages, where its seed-like fruits are scattered between folds of woollen clothes to preserve them against insect attack.

The plant is a stimulant, carminative, diuretic.

In laboratory findings, black cumin has shown surprising results. Its alcoholic extracts have exhibited anti-implantation effect. They also showed anti-bacterial activity against *E. Coli* and

Micrococcus species. They have been found to cause analgesic and antifertility actions.

The Profile

Botanical Name	:	*Nigella sativa* L.
English Name	:	Black Cumin.
Indian Names	:	Bengali : *Kalijira*
		Hindi, Punjabi
		& Urdu : *Kalaunji, Kalajira*
		Malayalam : *Karumshiragam*
		Marathi : *Kalanjire*
		Sanskrit : *Krishna-Jiraka*
		Tamil : *Karunjiragam*
		Telugu : *Nulajilakara*
Family	:	Ranunculaceae.
Appearance	:	A small herb, often cultivated. Leaves, long and linear. Flowers, pale blue. Seeds, black, trigonous.
Distribution	:	Cultivated in Punjab, Himachal Pradesh, Bengal, Assam and Bihar.
Medicinal Parts	:	Seeds.

In Tradition

AILMENT	PRESCRIPTION
❧ Gout, lumbago, rheumatism	: Take equal quantity of asparagus seeds (*Shatavari*), black cumin seeds, fenugreek seeds and ajwain. Powder. Take $1/2$ tsp of this powder every morning.

❧ Hiccups : Take $1/2$ tsp powder of black cumin seeds with a glass of buttermilk.

❧ Intestinal worms and parasites : Take $1/2$ tsp powder of black cumin seeds along with rice-gruel.

❧ Piles : Take 1 tbsp black cumin seeds and roast them. Mix in another tbsp black cumin seeds (unroasted). Now grind both together into a very fine powder. Take $1/2$ tsp of this mixture along with a glass of water.

❧ Renal colic (Kidney-pain) : Grind 2 tbsp black cumin seeds, 1 tbsp ajwain and 1 tsp black salt along with a little vinegar into a fine paste. Take a 1 tsp dose frequently.

❧ Fever, intermittent fever, venereal diseases : Soak some nirgundi leaves (*Vitex negundo*) in drinking water kept in a mud pot. Take a glass of this water and add $1/2$ tsp powdered black cumin seeds and drink.

❧ Headache, swellings in the body : Grind black cumin seeds with a little hot water and apply on affected parts.

❧ Acne of face, alopecia, leucoderma, ringworm : Grind some black cumin seeds with a little vinegar to a smooth paste. Apply on affected parts.

❧ Boils and pustules : Grind some black cumin seeds in a little water and apply the paste on affected areas.

✤ Leucoderma : Grind 1 tsp black cumin seeds in 1 tsp vinegar and apply.

✤ Skin-diseases : Fry 1 tsp black cumin in 1 tbsp coconut oil till it is charred. Allow it to cool and apply on the affected areas.

✤ Skin-infections : Grind black cumin seeds into a fine paste. Mix in 1 tsp sesame oil. Apply on affected areas.

✤ Amnesia, dullness of memory : Take $1/2$ tsp black cumin powder and mix it with honey. Eat small quantities twice a day.

✤ Aphrodisiac : Take a few drops of oil of black cumin with betel leaf.

✤ Toxin due to animal-bite, dog-bite, etc : Take $1/2$ tsp powder of black cumin seeds twice daily.

✤ Yellow pigmentation in eyes, as a result of jaundice : Grind $1/4$ tsp black cumin seeds in breast milk and introduce a pinch into the nostrils.

Note: Individual results may vary.

In Science

Eckey, E. W. 1954. *Vegetable Fats and Oils*. New York: Reinhold Publishing Corporation. (On *Nigella* oil.)

Hoppe, H. A. 1958. *Drogenkunde: Handbuck der Pflanzlic Tierischen Rohstoffe.* 7th edn. Hamburg: Cram de Gruyer & Co.

Hasan, C. M. et al. 1992. *In-vitro* anti-bacterial screening of the oils of *Nigella sativa* seeds. *Bangladesh J. Botany* 18(2) 171–174. (*Nigella* oil effective against gram-positive and gram-negative bacteria.)

Khanna, T. et al. 1990. Some CNS and analgesic activity of *Nigella sativa* (*kalonji*) oil. (Abstract) *Conf. Pharmacol. Syrup. Herbal Drugs.* New Delhi. p. 4. (Analgesic activity of *Nigella* oil.)

Kirtikar, K. R. and B. D. Basu. 1935. *Indian Medicinal Plants.* 4 vols. 2nd edn. Revised by E. Blatter et al. Allahabad: Lalit Mohan Basu. (*Nigella* occupies a special place among Indian herbs.)

Wehmer, C. 1935. *Die Pflazenstoffe,* Verlag von Gustav Fischer Jena. 2 vols. 1929–1931; Suppl. 1935. (Role of *Nigella*.) (In German)

29

Tulsi

Ocimum sanctum

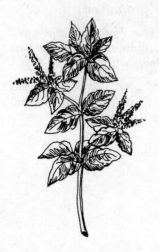

Tulsi, like ambrosia rose from the churning of the ocean and like ambrosia, it is to be sought after and cherished.

—The Puranas

Holy Life Preserver

Holy basil, popularly called tulsi, is a mystic plant of India, closely linked to the very roots of her civilisation.

The plant is worshipped every day by orthodox Hindus. It is widely believed to possess miraculous properties that destroy all kinds of evils.

It is also believed that due to its influence one escapes sudden and untimely death.

Not only Indians, but people elsewhere too revere this plant.

Haitian shopkeepers sprinkle basil water over their places of business to chase away evil spirits and to bring buyers prosperity.

In rural New Mexico, carrying basil in the pocket or purse is supposed to attract money into them. Further, a woman who wishes to stop her husband philandering is made to go through a ritual of dusting basil powder over her breasts.

Science has endorsed that tulsi can cure mental stress and enhance physical endurance. In most of the Hindu temples, tulsi-soaked water is distributed to devotees to cure their stress: physical, mental or spiritual.

The profile

Botanical Names	: *Ocimum tenuiflorum* Linn. *Ocimum sanctum* Linn.
English Name	: Holy Basil.
Indian Names	: Bengali, Gujarati, Hindi and Telugu : *Tulsi* Kannada : *Vishnu Tulasi* Malayalam : *Trittavu* Marathi : *Tulshi* Sanskrit : *Manjari, Krishna Tulsi* Tamil : *Tulasi*
Family	: Lamiaceae.
Appearance	: Erect, aromatic, hairy sub-shrub; flowers, small, purplish.
Distribution	: Common in plains, mostly in home yards. The plant is also found in the neighbouring countries.
Medicinal Parts	: Leaves, seeds, roots, extracts.
Preparation	: *Infusion:* Steep 1 tsp dried herb in $1/2$ cup water. Can be sweetened with honey, if taken for cough. Decoction, paste (of fresh leaves), powder (of dried leaves).

In Tradition

AILMENT	PRESCRIPTION
☙ Liver problems	: Clean 10–15 leaves in hot water and eat every morning. Wash it down with a glass of hot water.
☙ Colic	: Grind 1 tbsp tulsi leaves in water to make a fine paste and apply around the navel and on the abdomen.
☙ Digestion problems, dysentery, gastro-enteritis, gas problem, stomach ache	: A decoction of 15–20 tulsi leaves taken along with a pinch of rock salt.
☙ Harmless preparation for stomach trouble, especially in children	: Take 1/4 tsp seed paste with 1 teacup milk.
☙ Fever, malarial fever	: Grind equal quantities of bel flower and tulsi leaves and extract the juice. Take 1 tsp with 1 tsp honey.
☙ Fevers caused by *pitta*-aggravation	: Boil 20 leaves with 1 tsp crushed ginger in 1 teacup water, reduced to half a cup. Take 2 or 3 times a day.
☙ Fevers of unknown origin	: Boil 1 tbsp leaves with 1 tsp powdered cardamom in 2 teacups water. Take 1 cup of this decoction with milk and sugar to taste, 2 or 3 times a day.

❧ Toxic fever : Take 51 big tulsi leaves. Mix with 21 peppercorns and make a paste. Roll into small pills of the size of a grain of pepper. One such pill is to be taken once in the evening.

❧ Prophylactic malaria : A decoction of 15–20 tulsi leaves taken along with 1/2 tsp pepper powder.

❧ Ear diseases : Leaf juice used as ear drops.

❧ Headache : Grind 10–15 leaves with four cloves and 1 tsp dried ginger into a fine paste and apply on forehead.

: Finely ground leaf powder, snuffed occasionally.

❧ Cold, stomach upset : Boil 10–15 leaves in water and drink.

❧ Cold and cough : Juice of leaves (10–15) with 1 tsp each juices of ginger, betel leaf and honey.

: Tulsi leaves (15–20), frequently chewed with jaggery.

❧ Chest diseases, fever due to T.B. : Boil 20 leaves in 2 teacups water, reduced to 1 cup. Add to this 1 tsp sugar candy and 2 tsp honey. Take 2 tbsp 2 or 3 times a day.

❧ Prevention of cold : 10 leaves boiled in 1 teacup cow's milk. This is a recommended nutritive supplement for children.

❧ Insect bite : Take 1 tsp leaf juice and drink with water. Also apply externally.

❧ Ringworm : Grind finely a bunch of leaves and apply on the cleaned affected area.

❧ Skin diseases : Take 1 tsp juice of tulsi leaves every day. Also apply externally.

❧ Aphrodisiac : Take $1/2$ tsp powdered root with 1 tsp ghee.

❧ Cardiac pain, cold, influenza, low blood pressure, pain in ribs, skin diseases, worms, urinary diseases : Juice of leaves (10–15) mixed with 1 tsp honey.

❧ Longevity, rejuvenation : 5 to 10 leaves taken along with water every morning on an empty stomach continuously for 108 days.

❧ Unpleasant body odour : Soak 10–15 tulsi leaves in 1 teacup water and eat every morning for a month. (*Note:* avoid meat and foods rich in protein.)

Note: Individual results may vary.

A Word of Caution

Tulsi, in excess, may impair sperm-production as it possesses significant antifertility and abortifacient properties.

The Plucking Ritual

Indian civilization regards plants as living beings.

Long before scientists like Sir. J. C.Bose and several others could scientifically demonstrate that plants are as sensitive as human beings and they do have emotion, the ancient Indian customs and traditions had acknowledged it.

The traditional codes prescribe that plants should not be indiscriminately injured. While plucking flowers, fruits, bark, etc one should exercise great care and caution. One should not be violent or indifferent towards the hapless plants. One should exhibit awareness of their sensitivities.

Before plucking any portion of the plant, it should be first watered and caressed. Then, by uttering the name of the Almighty (e.g. 'Krishna, Krishna' in the case of tulsi, Krishna being the lord whose favourite is tulsi) and seeking the blessings of the plant-spirit in alleviating the problem for which the plant is plucked, only the required quantity of the plant-part should be taken out.

Normally, it is advised not to pluck any part of the plant after sunset to maintain tranquillity.

In Science

Batta, S. K. and G. Santhakumari. 1971. Antifertility effect of *Ocimum sanctum* and *Hibiscus rosa-sinensis*. *Indian J. Med. Res.* 59(5):771–781. (Abortifacient properties of tulsi.)

Bhargava, K. P. and N. Singh. 1981. Anti-stress activity of *Ocimum sanctum* Linn. *Indian J. Med. Res.* 73:443. (Tulsi's anti-stress properties.)

Bhat, J. V. and R. Broker. 1953. Action of some plant extracts on pathogenic *Staphylococci*. *J. Sci. Industr. Res.* 12:540–542. (Tulsi's anti-bacterial properties.)

Chopra, R. N. et al. 1956. *Glossary of Indian Medicinal Plants.* 179. New Delhi: Council of Scientific and Industrial Research. (Liver-protective, anti-malarial and anti-stress action of tulsi.)

Das, S. K. et al. 1983. Tulsi in the treatment of viral encephalitis. *Antiseptic* 80(7):323–327.

Gupta, K. C. and R. Viswanathan. 1955. *Antib. and Chem.* 51:22. (The oil obtained from *Ocimum sanctum* by ether extraction acted significantly on *M. tuberculosis.*)

Grover, G. S. and J. T. Rao. 1977. Investigations on the anti-microbial efficiency of essential oils from *Ocimum sanctum* and *Ocimum gratissimum. Perfum. und Kosmef.* 58(11):326–328. (Tulsi's essential oil exhibits anti-microbial effect; it was found active against fungi like *Aspergillus niger, R. stolonifer* and *Penicillium digitatum.*)

Hartwel, J. L. 1969. Plants used against cancer: a survey. *Lloydia* 32:247.

Joshi, C. G and N. G. Nagar. 1952. Antibiotic activity of some Indian medicinal plants. *J. Sci. Industr. Res.* 11B(6):261. (Ether fraction of tulsi leaves shows activity against bacteria *S. aureus* and *E. coli.*)

Kasinathan, S. et al. 1972. Antifertility effect of *Ocimum sanctum* Linn. *Indian J. Exptl. Biol.* 10(1):23–25 (Male mice treated with the tulsi-drug failed to fertilize the proven fertile female mice; tulsi also caused mild impairment of sperm-production.)

Mandal, S. et al. 1993. *Ocimum sanctum* L. A Study of gastric ulceration and gastric secretion in rats. *Indian J. Physiol. & Pharmacol.* 37(1):91–92. (Tulsi-extract has anti-ulcerogenic property against experimental ulcers.)

Matsubiro, A. and D. Nakada. 1955. Short Note on anti-tubercular substances of tulsi. *Antibiotic Chemotherapy* 5(22): *Chem. Abstr.* 1955 49:6368d. (A chemical study relating to the anti-tubercular principle obtained from tulsi.)

Palit, G. et al. 1983. An experimental evaluation of anti-asthmatic plant drugs from ancient Ayurvedic medicine. *Aspects Allergy Immunol.* 16:36. (Alcoholic extract of tulsi leaves exhibited dose-dependent protection against asthma in guinea pigs. The results confirm its use in bronchial asthma.)

Rajalakshmi, G. et al. 1988. Role of tulasi (*Ocimum sanctum* Linn) in the management of *Manjal Kamalai* (Viral Hepatitis). *Jour. Res. Ayur. Sid.* IX, 3–4:118–123. (The plant showed highly significant clinical and bio-chemical clearance of the viral disease in 14 days treatment.)

Reddi, G. S. et al. 1986. Chemotherapy of tuberculosis—Anti-tubercular activity of tulsi leaf extract. *Filoterapia* 57:114.

Roy, A. N. et al. 1979. The inhibitory effect of plant juices on the infectivity of top necrosis virus of pea. *Indian J. Microbiol.* 19:198. (Anti-stress and anti-viral activity of juice of tulsi leaves against Top-necrosis virus.)

Sarkar, A. et al. 1994. Changes in blood-lipid profile after administration of *Ocimum sanctum* (tulsi) leaves in the normal albino rabbits. *Indian J. Physiol. Pharmacol.* 38(4):311–312. (Tulsi purifies the blood.)

Seethalakshmi, B. et al. 1981. Protective effect of *Ocimum sanctum* in experimental liver injury in albino rats. *Proc. Indian Pharmacol. Soc. XIV Ann. Conf. Bombay,* Dec 29–31,1981; *Indian J. Pharmacol.* 14:63. (The plant exhibited enhancement of physical endurance and prevention of stress induced gastric ulcers; it also afforded protection against hepatotoxicity in mice and rats.)

Sen, P. et al. 1992. Mechanism of anti-stress activity of *Ocimum sanctum* Linn. eugenol and *Tinospora malabarica* in experimental animals. *Indian J. Exp. Biol.* 30(7):592–596.

Seth, S. D. et al. 1981. Antispermatogenic effect of *Ocimum sanctum*. *Indian J. Exptl. Biol.* 19:975. (Impairment in sperm production is reported in benzene-extract of leaves; the weight of testes and sperm-count were also reduced.)

Sharma, R. et al. 1987. Management of tropical pulmonary eosinophilia in children with Ayurvedic drugs. *Jour. of Res. and Edn. in Ind. Med.* 6(1–2):11–17.

Singh, N. et al. 1977. Experimental evaluation of adaptogenic properties of *Ocimum sanctum*. *Indian Pharmacological Society Proc.* 74. (Anti-stress agent in tulsi.)

Singh, N. et al. 1979. Experimental evaluation of anti-stress (adaptogenic) effects of some plant drugs. XII *Ann. Conf. Indian Pharmacological Society Proc.* 63. (Tulsi's action evaluated.)

Singh, S. P. et al. 1983. Antifungal activity of essential oils of some *Labiatae* plants against dermatophytes. *Indian Perfum.* 27:171. (Antifungal activity of tulsi.)

Singh, T. J. et al. 1970. Preliminary pharmacological investigations of *Ocimum sanctum* Linn. *Indian J. Pharm.* 32(4):92–94. (Antispasmodic activity of tulsi.)

Vijayalakshmi, K. et al. 1979. Nematicidal properties of some indigenous plant materials against second stage juveniles of *Meloidogene incognita* (Kaffoid and white) Chitwood. *Indian J. Entomol.* 41:326. (Water extract of tulsi destroyed the plant parasite nematode.)

30

Khuskhus

Papaver somniferum

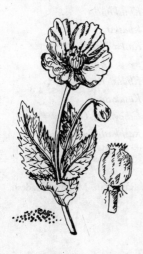

*Khuskhus ensures brightness,
energy and strength.*

—Raaja Nighantu

Non-addictive Medicine from the Poppy

The harmless poppy-seeds which are used in the kitchen come from a powerful plant, the plant which produces the opium drug.

Khuskhus seeds are so tiny that about a thousand of them weigh hardly 0.4 g! Yet they play an important role as a highly nutritive food-stuff and as medicine.

In traditional medicine, khuskhus is used to fight obstinate constipation and in catarrh of the bladder. A fatty oil extracted from the seeds, besides finding its way into the kitchen, is also used for treating diarrhoea, dysentery and scalds.

The Profile

Botanical Name	:	*Papaver somniferum* L.
English Name	:	Opium Poppy.
Indian Names	:	Bengali,
		Hindi,
		Punjabi &
		Urdu : *Kaskash*
		Gujarati : *Khuskhush*
		Kannada : *Khasksi*
		Malayalam : *Kasha Kasha*
		Marathi : *Khus Khus*
		Sanskrit : *Khasa, Khakasa*
		Tamil : *Kasakasa*
		Telugu : *Gasagasla, Gasalu.*
		Urdu : *Kashkash Sufaid*
Family	:	Papaveraceae.
Distribution	:	Uttar Pradesh, Rajasthan, Madhya Pradesh.
Medicinal Parts	:	Seeds.

In Tradition

AILMENT	PRESCRIPTION
✦ Haemophilia	: Add more khuskhus to your normal diet (in the form of chutneys, curries, sweet dishes, etc).
✦ Burning eyes, dandruff	: Grind an onion with 1 tsp each black pepper and 1/2 teacup khuskhus in milk. Apply this paste on the head.

Allow it to dry for 15–20 mts. Wash in warm water.

❧ Sexual debility : Mix 1 tsp each wheat grains, fenugreek seeds and khuskhus and soak in water overnight. Grind into a fine paste. To this paste add milk and sugar to taste. Take every day for a few days continuously.

❧ Cough : Boil 2 tsp khuskhus and 3 tsp cut liquorice root in 1 teacup water for 10 mts. Strain and drink, twice daily.

❧ Dry itch in body, certain types of skin-allergies : Grind 1 tbsp khuskhus with 1 tsp water. Add 1 tsp lime juice. Apply on the affected areas.

❧ Prickly heat : Grind finely 1 tbsp each khuskhus, tender neem leaves and goat's milk and apply on the affected areas.

❧ Insomnia : 1 tbsp each khuskhus and *Cannabis* leaves commonly used in the preparation of bhang are ground with a little water and applied on soles and palms before going to bed.

❧ Physical weakness, sexual debility : Fry in 1 tbsp butter 2 tsp each wheat flour, almond paste and khuskhus paste. Eat this along with 1 teacup boiled leaves of fenugreek.

207

❧ Insomnia : Blend about 10 soaked almonds with 1 tbsp khuskhus in milk. Smear this paste on soles and palms before going to bed.

: Boil $1/2$ tsp each khuskhus and lettuce seeds in 1 teacup water. Strain and sweeten with 1 tsp honey. Twice daily.

Note: Individual results may vary.

A Word of Caution

Excess use of khuskhus heats up the system. According to some authors, it may have a sedative effect as well.

Khuskhus is not to be confused with *khaskhas* or vetiver (*Vetiveria• zizanoides*), a perennial grass whose dried roots yield as essential oil, popular in perfumery, cosmetics and for flavouring sherbets.

In Science

Chopra, R. N. et al. 1949. *Poisonous Plants of India.* Calcutta: Government Press.

Hunter, H. and H. M. Leake. 1933. *Recent Advances in Agricultural Plant Breeding.* London: J&A Churchill Ltd. (Breeding poppy for opium alkaloids.)

Modi, J. P. 1945. *A Text-book of Medical Jurisprudence and Toxicology.* Bombay: Tripathi Ltd.

Mollison, J. 1901. *A Text-book of Indian Agriculture.* 3 vols. Bombay: Government of Bombay. (Cultivation of opium poppy in India.)

Mukerji, N. G. 1915. *Hand-book of Indian Agriculture.* 3rd edn. Calcutta: Thacker, Spink & Co. (Horticulture and the opium poppy.)

Snell, F. D. and C. T. Snell. 1952. *Chemicals of Commerce.* 2nd edn. D. van Nostrand & Co. Inc. (Opium alkaloids and their properties.)

Steinmetz, E. F. 1954. *Materia Medica Vegetabilis.* 3 vols. Holland. (Opium as a medicine.)

Wehmer, C. 1935. *Die Pflanzenstoffe.* Jena: Verlag von Gustav Fischer. 2 vols. 1929–1931; Suppl. 1935. (On opium and its alkaloids.) (In German)

Winton, A. L. and K. B. Winton. 1935. *The Structure and Composition of Foods.* New York: John Wiley & Sons. (Poppy seeds as a foodstuff.)

31

Amla
Phyllanthus emblica

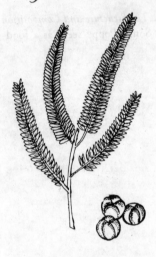

One can survive by consuming the fruit juice of amalaki only.

—Vamana Purana, *91.51.*
(2nd Century A.D.)

A Taste of Amla

In Ayurvedic medicine, taste is all-important. Different food-materials are categorized according to the six defined tastes: sweet, sour, salty, bitter, pungent and astringent.

A correct balancing of these tastes is considered essential for the growth of a healthy body. In other words, a healthy diet has to contain a combination of all six tastes.

Herbs such as emblic myrobalan (popularly known in India as amla) cater to all the six tastes at one go. They act on the body to increase or decrease the three humours: *kapha*, *pitta* and *vata.*

Fully recognizing its importance, the Hindus associate it with the mythological Lord of Wealth, Kubera. It is also referred to as *dhatri,* the nurse. It rejuvenates the body cells, tones up the tissues and strengthens the organs. It is believed to increase the life-energy (*prana*) and has a *sattvic* (soothing) effect on the mind.

There are two varieties of amla: the wild one with small fruits and the cultivated one, called Banarsi, with bigger fruits. Both are known to possess medicinal value.

Almost all parts of this plant are of great medicinal use in the traditional systems of medicine: leaves, flowers, fruits, seeds, roots and bark. Of them, fruits constitute the more significant drug.

Storehouse of Vitamin C

Being the cheapest and at the same time, the richest source of Vitamin C, dried amla provides as much as 3000 mg of Vitamin C per 100 g, which is heat-stable, i.e. not denatured by boiling. Scientific studies have further indicated that Vitamin C here is more easily assimilated into the human system as compared to the other synthetic sources.

Amla is one of the Three Great Myrobalans extensively used in the traditional systems of Ayurveda and Siddha and also in the Tibetan school of medicine. Emblic in combination with the other two myrobalans, chebulic and belleric forms the formidable *Triphala*, considered to be of key medicinal importance.

Amla *per se* is a *kaya kalpa.* It imparts youthful vigour, strengthens lungs and cures excessive thirst, burning sensation, vomiting, diabetes, emaciation, anorexia, toxicity, fever, impurity of blood and haemorrhage. It activates the liver, pancreas, circulatory system and digestive system. It is diuretic, astringent, digestive, aphrodisiac, laxative and tonic. It is a coolant for the human engine.

For the beauty-conscious, like lime, amla also works wonders: it tightens up sagging skin and guards against flabbiness and wrinkles.

211

The Profie

Botanical Names	: *Phyllanthus emblica* L.
	Emblica officinalis Gaertn.
English Names	: Emblic, Emblic Myrobalan.

Indian Names	:		
		Assamese	: *Chukna Amlaki*
		Bengali	: *Amloki*
		Gujarati	: *Amran*
		Hindi	: *Amla (Aonla)*
		Malayalam	: *Amlakam*
		Marathi	: *Amla*
		Oriya	: *Aora*
		Sanskrit	: *Amlika*
		Tamil	: *Nellikka*

Family	: Euphorbiaceae.
Appearance	: A medium tree with smooth greenish-grey exfoliating bark. Leaves feathery. Fruits globose pale-green, 1 to 5 cm. in diameter, fleshy, sour in taste, 6-lobed.
Distribution	: Throughout tropical and sub-tropical India, upto 1500 m. Found in plenty in the Madhya Pradesh forests.
Medicinal Parts	: Fruits, leaves, flowers, seeds, roots, bark.

In Tradition

AILMENT	PRESCRIPTION
✤ Diarrhoea	: Grind 1 tsp leaf buds into a very fine paste. Add 1 teacup buttermilk. Drink 2 or 3 times a day.

212

❧ Constipation : Soak 1 or 2 dried fruits in water overnight. Mash and filter the next morning. Add 1 tsp honey and drink.

❧ Urinary problems : Soak separately 2 tsp each dried amla and raisins in water overnight. Mash, filter and drink the next morning. Continue for a few days.

❧ Dandruff,
eye-problems,
hair-loss, jaundice,
night blindness,
pitta-aggravation

: Crush fresh amla fruits along with a little water and express about 2 teacups juice. Add to this equal quantities of cow's milk and juice of trailing eclipta. Add 8 teacups coconut water and 6 teacups sesame oil. Mix in 3 tsp each fine powder of the following separately:

: Liquorice, wild turmeric, nutmeg, mace, chebulic myrobalan, belleric myrobalan, dried ginger and black pepper. Now mix all the ingredients together in a vessel and heat over low flame. When the mixture reduces in volume and loses all traces of moisture, leaving behind a thick oil, remove from the fire. Allow it to cool. Bottle. Take 2 to 3 tsp of this oil twice a week and apply on scalp. Massage with fingers for 10 minutes. Wash it off with water.

❧ Headache,
heaviness in head
: Grind the fresh fruits into a fine paste and apply on affected parts.

❧ Mouth ulcers : Take 1 tsp finely powdered root bark and mix with honey. Apply on affected areas frequently.

213

❧ Skin-problems : Grind the dried fruits into a fine powder and use as a substitute for soap.

❧ Memory loss : Mix 1 tsp each root powder and white sesame seed powder. Add 1 tsp honey and eat every day for a few days.

❧ Aggravation of *pitta*, dyspnoea, fever, leucorrhoea, menorrhagia, nausea, *vata* and *kapha*—early stages : Clean, dry and powder 1 tsp of the root. Boil in 1 cup water till it is reduced to $1/2$ cup. And a little sugar and drink on an empty stomach every morning.

❧ Anxiety, body heat, diabetes, deficiency in blood, loss of appetite, nervousness, premature ejaculation, sexual debility : Remove seeds from fresh fruits and grind the pulp into a fine paste. Tie it in a muslin cloth and squeeze out the juice. Take 2 tsp of this juice and mix it with two teaspoonfuls each honey and lime juice. Add 1 teacup water and drink on an empty stomach every morning. Whenever fresh fruits are not available, dried amla can be used. Soak 1 tbsp the previous night in a cup of water. The following morning, add $1/8$ tsp finely ground black pepper powder and 2 tsp lime juice. Dilute it if necessary with water and drink every morning regularly on an empty stomach. (*Attention:* The treatment should continue for at least 120 days to achieve expected results.)

214

❖ Bone-fever, breathing problems, cancer, cough, gas, phlegm, TB, stomach problems

: Boil 2 teacups dried amla fruits in 4 teacups water till the volume is reduced to 1 teacup. In a separate vessel, make a sugar syrup by dissolving 1 teacup sugar in adequate water and heating it. Now mix the amla decoction with sugar syrup and heat over a low flame and stir the mixture frequently. Separately mix the finely ground powder of the following: 1 tbsp each dried ginger, black pepper and long pepper; 1 tsp each cloves, cardamom, sal, (*Shorea robusta*) liquorice, coriander seeds, cumin. Now, fold in the powder-mixture little by little into the boiling mixture while stirring. Allow it to be heated till the desired consistency is obtained. Now add 1 teacup ghee made from cow's milk, stir well and remove from fire. Once the mixture is cooled, it can be stored in a clean, dry glass bottle. Take 1 tsp mixture along with a little milk twice a day.

Note: Individual results may vary.

A Word of Caution

Some practitioners insist that whenever amla is used in cuisine or in medicine, one should avoid meat, sweets, tobacco and sex.

In Science

Aiyer, K. N. and M. Kolammal. 1963. *Pharmacognosy of Ayurvedic Drugs*. Nos. 4–9. Trivandrum.

Banu, N. et al. 1982. Role of *amalaki* (*Emblica officinalis*) rasayana in experimental peptic ulcer. *Sour. Res. Edn. Ind. Med.* 1(1):29–34. (Amla cures peptic ulcer.)

Chawla, Y. K. et al. 1987. Treatment of dyspepsia with *amalaki* (*Emblica officinalis* Linn.) an Ayurvedic drug. *Vagbhata* 5(3):24–26.

Dhar, D. C. et al. 1951. Chemical examination of the seed of *Emblica· officinalis* Gaertn. Part I—The fatty oil and its component fatty acids. *J. Sci. Industr. Res.* 10B:88–91. (A chemical examination.)

Dhar, D. C. et al. 1956. Studies on *Emblica officinalis* Gaertn. Part II—Chromatographic study of some constituents of Amla. *J. Sci. Industr. Res.* 15C:205–206.

Husain, S. J. 1975. *Screening of some unani cardiotonic drugs.* D.U.M. Thesis. Aligarh Muslim University.

Jain, S. K. 1968. *Medicinal Plants* 76. New Delhi. (A detail here: the leaves of amla are used as manure in cardamom plantations.)

Jamwal, K. S. et al. 1959. Pharmacological investigation of the fruit of *Emblica officinalis* Gaertn. *J. Sci. Industr. Res.* 18C:180–181.

Khurana, M. L. et al. 1960. Expectorant activity of *Emblica officinalis* Gaertn. *J. Scient. Ind. Res* 19C:60. (A study.)

Kurup, P. N. V. et al. 1979. *Handbook of Medicinal Plants.* New Delhi. (On a handful of medicinal plants including amla.)

Maroli, S and S. Javale. 1990. Amalaki *Phyllanthus emblica*—an Ayurvedic rejuvenator. *Pediatr. Clin. India* 17(2):42–44. (Effects of the fruit on digestive, nervous, cardio-vascular and reproductive systems.)

Shead, A. et al. 1992. Effect of *Phyllanthus* plant extracts on duck hepatitis B virus *in vitro* and *in vivo*. *Antiviral Res.* 18(2):127–138.

Singh, B. N. and P. V. Sharma 1971. Effect of *amalaki* on *amlapitta*. *Jour. Res. Ind. Med.* 5(2):223–230.

Summanen, J. et al. 1993. Anti-inflammatory activity of leaf-extract of *Emblica officinalis. Planta Med.* 59 (*Suppl.*) A 666. (Effect of amla leaves in reducing inflammation.)

Tariq, M. et al. 1977. Protective effects of fruit extracts of *Emblica officinalis* Gaertn. and *Terminalia belerica* Roxb. in experimental myocardinal necrosis in rats. *Indian J. Exp. Biol.* 15:485.

Thakur, C. P. and K. Mandal. 1984. Effect of *Emblica officinalis* in cholesterol-induced artherosclerosis in rabbits. *Ind J. Med. Res.* 79:142–146. (Amla's role in artherosclerosis.)

Thakur, C. P. 1985. *Emblica officinalis* reduces serum, aortic and hepatic cholesterol in rabbits. *Experientia 1985*, 41:423.

Yaqueenuddin, et al. 1990. Pharmacological evaluation of the anti-emetic action of *Emblica officinale* Gaertn. *Pakistan J. Sci. Indl. Res.* 33(7):268–269.

32

Pepper
Piper nigrum

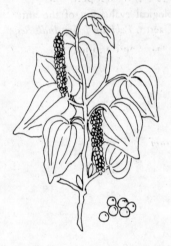

> *The bitter pepper is germicidal and loved by yavanas.*
>
> —Abhidaana Manjari

Sun Fruit

Pepper's medicinal value has been known to mankind from time immemorial.

It's name in Sanskrit, *Marich,* refers to the sun. The name is based on the belief that a very large dose of the sun's energy is trapped in the fruits of pepper. Being hot and pungent, it increases digestive power and improves appetite.

In addition to this, it can cure a host of diseases: cold, sinus congestion, cough, cardiac diseases, degenerated metabolism, colic, worms, diabetes, obesity, piles, dyspnoea, blood diseases, eczema, intermittent fevers, neurites, dysentery, night blindness, etc.

Black, White and Green

There are three varieties of pepper: black pepper, white pepper and green pepper.

While black pepper constitutes the dried but unripe fruits, white pepper is obtained from ripe fruits by removing their outer skin. Green pepper refers to the tender green spikes which are straightaway pickled in salt water for preservation and use.

Piperine, the main active principle of pepper, imparts its characteristic taste.

Clinical findings have confirmed pepper's traditional medicinal role. Piperine protects the liver and is analgesic and anti-inflammatory. It stimulates thyroid glands. It also shows CNS-depressant activity.

The Profile

Botanical Name	:	*Piper nigrum* L.
English Names	:	Pepper, Black Pepper, Common Pepper.
Indian Names	:	Bengali : *Gol Marich, Kalomarich*
		Gujarati : *Kala Mari, Kalomirich*
		Hindi and
		Punjabi : *Kali Mirch*
		Kannada : *Kare Menasu*
		Kashmiri : *Marutis*
		Malayalam : *Kurumulaku*
		Marathi : *Mire, Kali Mirch*
		Oriya : *Gol Maricha*
		Sanskrit : *Maricha Ushana, Hopusha*
		Tamil : *Milagu*
		Telugu : *Miriyalu*
		Urdu : *Siah Mirch*
Family	:	Piperaceae.
Appearance	:	The plant is an evergreen creeper.

219

| Distribution | : Widely cultivated in various parts of India, mainly in South India. Kerala alone contributes ninety-six per cent of the total production in the country. |
| Medicinal Parts | : Fruits. |

In Tradition

AILMENT	PRESCRIPTION
✤ Rheumatic pains	: 2 to 3 tsp pepper powder is fried in 2 tsp seasame oil until charred. When it is warm, it is applied on the affected areas.
✤ Arthritis	: Combine 6 tsp each dried ginger and caraway seeds and 3 tsp black pepper and grind into a very fine powder and preserve. *Dose*: $1/2$ tsp with water thrice daily.
✤ Digestive disorders, lack of appetite	: $1/2$ tsp ground pepper mixed with 1 tbsp jaggery powder to be taken.
✤ Indigestion	: Grind 3 tsp pepper with 6 tsp each ginger and caraway seeds into a fine powder and preserve. Take $1/2$ tsp with water twice daily.
✤ Indigestion, heaviness in stomach	: $1/4$ tsp each pepper powder and cumin powder is mixed in 1 teacup buttermilk. Drink this a few times.
✤ Cold, fever	: $1/2$ tsp ground pepper is mixed in warm water along with 1 tsp palm candy. This drink is taken at bedtime.

❧ Bad breath, bleeding gums, gum inflammation, pus formation in gums, pyorrhoea

: A mixture of equal quantities of fine salt and pepper powder, thoroughly massaged over the gums.

❧ Cataract

: Grind 7 black peppercorns with 7 almond kernels into a fine paste, mix in some milk and sugar candy. Sift and drink everyday. (*Note*: This treatment helps the eyes regain normalcy.)

: Grind 2 tsp white pepper along with 5 tsp almond kernels, and 3 tsp cane sugar (unrefined). Mix in 2 tsp ghee. *Dose*: 2 tsp twice daily for one month. (*Note:* This treatment prevents the increasing opacity of the cornea.)

❧ Headache

: Grind 5 corns of black pepper, 3 tsp each lavender flowers and coriander seeds into a fine powder. Take one-half of this with water early in the morning, then take rest.

❧ Headache, epileptic seizures, sinus congestion

: Heat $1/4$ tsp pepper powder in $1/2$ tsp ghee. When cooled, use as nasal drops. (*Caution:* Pepper burns!)

❧ Toothache

: A mixture of finely powdered pepper and clove oil is applied on the affected areas.

❧ Dry cough, throat irritation

: $1/4$ tsp pepper powder is mixed with equal quantities of powder of caraway seeds and a pinch of common salt. This mixture is eaten frequently.

❧ Reproductive weakness, sexual debility
: Boil 1 teacup milk with $1/2$ tsp pepper powder and 6 to 8 crushed almonds. Take at bedtime.

❧ Common cold
: Boil 5 black pepper corns, 1 tsp wheat husk and $1/6$ tsp salt for 3 mts and strain. Take twice daily.

❧ Boils, inflamed surfaces as in urticaria and erysipelas
: Heat pepper powder in $1/2$ tsp ghee until charred. Use this as ointment. (*Caution*: Pepper burns!)

❧ Pimples
: Grind equal quantities of nutmeg, black pepper and sandalwood and apply frequently.

Note: Individual results may vary.

A Word of Caution

Pepper intake is not advisable for those who have inflammatory conditions of the digestive organs.

Pepper should be avoided by those who are prone to high *pitta* conditions as it heats up the body.

In excess, pepper can act as an irritant as its quality is *rajasic*.

In Science

Koul, I. B. and A. Kapil. 1993. Evaluation of the liver-protective potential of piperine, an active principle of black and long peppers. *Planta Med.* 59(5):413–417. (Piperine protects the liver.)

Lee, E. B. et al. 1984. Pharmacological study on piperine. *Arch. Pharma. Res.* 7(2):127–132. (Various pharmacological activities of piperine such as CNS depressant activity, analgesic, antipyretic and anti-inflammatory activities documented.)

Sethi, S. C. and J. S. Agarwal. 1952. Stabilization of Edible Fats by Spices and Condiments. Part I. *J. Sci. Industr. Res.* 11B:46. (Black pepper effectively checks the development of rancidity in vegetable oils.)

Sharma, M. L. et al. 1962. Chemische Untersuchungen des pfefferschaelnols (*Piper nigrum* L. Fam. Piperaceae) *Parfum u Kosmetik* 43:505–506. (In German.)

Sridharan, K. et al. 1978. Chemical and pharmacological screening of *Piper nigrum* L. leaves. *J. Res. Indian Med. Yoga.* 13:107–108. (Pepper: Its chemical composition and pharmacological value.)

Tripathi, S. N. and C. M. Tripathi. 1992 Clinical and experimental evaluation of endocrine response of herbal drugs. *Jour. Res. Ayur. Sid.* XIII, 3–4:174–178. (Black pepper showed significant stimulation of the thyroid gland.)

33

Almond
Prunus amygdalus

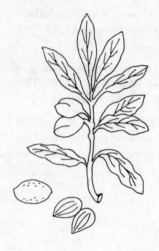

Almond renders beauty.

—Aatanga Samgraham

Amandin, an Ideal Milk Supplement

There is a common misconception that vegetarian food lacks protein.

Almond explodes all such myths as it contains twenty per cent protein—a percentage one finds hardly anywhere else in the plant kingdom. Leave alone the quantity, the quality of the protein is such that it is very easily digested. Its digestibility co-efficient is rated very high (ninety-four per cent) at nine per cent level intake.

The chief protein in almond is a globulin called amandin. It is considered to be a good supplement for milk.

For the ancient Greeks, the almond was a symbol of love and truth. They believed in its supernatural powers.

The Chinese were cultivating it as early as the 10th century B.C.

The ancient Europeans were aware of the medicinal and cosmetic importance of almonds.

Almond forms an ideal food for diabetics as it contains little or no carbohydrates. It is valuable in diets for peptic ulcers. The unripe fruit is used as an astringent application for the gums and mouth. For elders and growing children it is an ideal tonic.

In order to enhance its assimilation, almonds are often taken in combination with other spices like black pepper, khuskhus, turmeric, cardamom, etc.

Almond oil is somewhat like olive oil, but is hardly used in food because of its high price. Its principal uses are however, in the cosmetic and pharmaceutical industries.

The Profile

Botanical Names	:	*Prunus dulcis* (Miller) D.A. Webb. *Prunus amygdalus* Batsch *Prunus communis* (L) Arcang *Amygdalus communis* L.
English Name	:	Almond.
Indian Names	:	Bengali, Hindi, Marathi &
		Punjabi : *Badam*
		Kannada : *Badami*
		Malayalam : *Vatam Kotta*
		Tamil : *Vaadumai, Vaadamkottai*
		Telugu : *Badam Vittulu*
Appearance	:	A tree growing to the height of around 9 metres.
Family	:	A native of the Eastern Mediterranean, the almond is cultivated in Kashmir and the Punjab for its edible seeds.
Medicinal Parts	:	Kernel, oil, shell.

225

In Tradition

AILMENT	PRESCRIPTION
✤ Sprain	: Mix equal parts of almond oil and garlic oil and massage over the affected parts.
✤ Angina pectoris	: Thoroughly mix 2 tsp almond oil with 1 tsp rose oil. Rub gently on the chest morning and evening.
✤ Constipation	: Grind separately 5 tsp almonds and 5 tsp dried dates. Combine them and add 10 tsp honey. Take 3 tsp of this mixture twice daily.
✤ Constipation, cough, throat-irritation	: Soak 2–3 almonds and dried figs for a few hours in 1 teacup water. Remove the outer skin of the almonds and grind together to a paste. Add 1 tbsp honey and eat before going to bed.
✤ Kidney and liver malfunctioning	: Add more almonds to the daily diet.
✤ Early stages of cataract (This treatment helps eyes regain normal conditions and relieves hoarseness of throat.)	: Soak 8 to 10 almonds overnight in 1 teacup water. After discarding the outer skin, grind the kernels with 8 to 10 black peppercorns in 1 teacup water. Sift it and drink after adding sugar candy to taste. Once a day.
✤ Lice	: Grind 7 to 8 kernels with 1 to 2 tsp lime juice and apply on the hair.

❧ Falling hair : Apply a little almond oil on scalp frequently and massage.

❧ Wounds or lesions inside the nostrils : Drop 1 to 2 drops of almond oil into the nose.

❧ Yellowing of teeth, toothache, gum diseases : Burn the shells of almonds and powder. Use as toothpowder.

❧ Nervous weakness, sexual debility : Soak 8 to 10 almonds for a few hours and remove the outer skin. Grind the kernels along with 8 to 10 black peppercorns into a very thin paste. Mix into 1 teacup milk and take daily.

❧ Sexual debility : Make paranthas with a mixture of $1/2$ tsp each boiled fenugreek leaves, almonds, khuskhus and ghee and eat every day for 40 days.

: Cut and boil a few drumstick fruits and collect their pulp. Grind a few almonds and 2–3 pinches of saffron along with this pulp and eat every day for 40 days.

❧ Sexual under-development in women; undue delay in menstruation : 6 to 8 almonds, crushed and mixed in 1 teacup milk along with 1 egg yolk, $1/2$ tsp sesame powder and 1 tsp honey. Take once or twice a day.

227

❧ Cough, throat-
irritation

: Sprinkle some salt water on almond
kernels and fry them. Chew 5 or 6 nuts
frequently.

❧ Dry cough
due to heat,
body heat

: Add 2 to 3 drops of almond oil to
pomegranate juice and drink.

❧ Dry cough,
cough due to
heat, body heat

: Add 1 or 2 drops of almond oil to a
glass of milk and drink.

❧ Psoriasis, skin
problems

: Powder a few almonds and boil
thoroughly in some water. Apply this
paste on affected areas and let it remain
overnight. Next morning wash it off
with water.

❧ Skin problems

: Massage the body frequently with
almond oil.

❧ To improve
complexion

: Mix equal quantities of almond oil and
honey and apply on the face.

❧ Helps in
maintaining the
complexion of the
skin in exposed
regions. (Darkness
of skin due to
long exposure to
sun gets light-
ened by this
treatment.)

: Soak 10 almonds overnight in water.
After discarding the outer skin, grind
the kernels along with 1 tsp milk
cream into a very fine paste. Mix this
with 1 tsp coconut oil. Apply daily
on exposed parts of body, i.e. face,
neck, forearms, legs, etc every day.

❧ Anaemia,
body heat, body
weakness, cough,
sexual debility

: Soak 8 to 10 almonds and 1 tsp rice
overnight. Remove the outer skin.
Grind into a fine paste. Mix in some
milk and a pinch of turmeric powder.
Boil and drink along with sugar candy
or palm sugar to taste.

❧ Aphrodisiac

: Make a soup of 5 tsp powdered
almonds along with 1 tbsp cream and
1 egg yolk and drink.

❧ Insomnia

: Grind blanched almonds (8 to 10)
along with 1 tsp khuskhus in $1/2$ teacup
milk and smear the paste on palms and
soles at bedtime.

❧ Obesity (Avoid
fatty food, ice-
cream, chocolates,
etc)

: Grind 6 to 7 blanched almonds,
1 tsp rice, 1 or 2 tbsp juice of banana
flower into a fine paste. Pour into this
some milk and drink every day for
40 days.

❧ To develop the
body and muscles

: Soak 2 almonds, 5 pista kernels and
1 tsp khuskhus in 1 cup cow's milk for
an hour. Grind and warm with more
milk and palmyrah candy. Take daily
for 3 months.

❧ Vertigo

: Mix 7 to 8 almonds with 7 to 8 kernels
of pumpkin seeds, 1 tsp khuskhus and
3 tbsp wheat. Soak in water overnight.
Next morning, remove the outer skin
of the almonds and grind together into
a fine paste. Heat separately 2 tsp ghee
and fry $1/2$ tsp cloves. Add the paste to
it along with some milk and boil the

whole mixture. Sweeten with sugar and
drink every day for a few days.

Note : Individual results may vary.

A Word of Caution

In summer months and in hot climatic zones, almond should be
consumed after removing its brown outer skin which has a
tendency to produce enormous heat in the body.

In Science

Bailey, L. H. 1947. *Standard Cyclopaedia of Horticulture.* Reprinted.
Vol III. New York: Macmillan. p. 2832. (On the scientific cultivation
of almond.)

Chandler, W. H. 1957. *Deciduous Orchards.* 3rd edn. London: Henry
Kimpton. p. 362–364.

Hill, A. F. 1952. *Economic Botany: A Text-book of Useful Plants and
Plant Products.* 2nd edn. New York: McGraw-Hill. p. 356.

Howes, F. N. 1949. *Nuts: Their production and everyday uses.* London:
Faber & Faber. p. 110–112.

Kuppuswamy, S. et al. 1958. *Proteins in foods.* New Delhi: ICMR.
Special Report Series no. 33. p 99–102. (Protein quality of almond.)

Sham Singh et al. 1963. *Fruit culture in India.* New Delhi: ICAR. p. 354.

Thapar, A. R. 1960. *Horticulture in the hill-regions of North India.*
Directorate of Extension. New Delhi: Min. Food & Agric. p. 115.
(A survey-report on almond.)

Winton, A. L. and K. B. Winton. 1935. *The Structure and composition
of Foods.* Wiley, I:480–485. (Nutritive wealth of almond.)

Zeilinski, Q. B. 1980. *Modern Systematic Pomology.* Iowa: W.M.C. Brown
& Co. Inc. p. 169 (Growing an almond tree.)

34

Pomegranate

Punica granatum

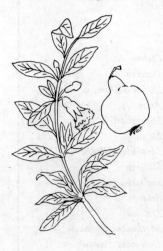

Flowers of anar are an ingredient of prescriptions for abortion.

—Hakeem H. Abdul Hameed Saheb

The Chinese Cure-All

What tulsi is to the Hindus, pomegranate is to the Chinese.

The pomegranate is grown practically in every Chinese household as it is believed to ward off the evil eye. Growing a tree in your garden is like having a pharmacy at your doorstep!

The rind has great medicinal properties. It is unfortunate that people who relish its pulp normally throw away this precious part of the fruit.

Besides the rind, other parts of this plant—flowers, stem-bark and fruit also have medicinal value.

Fresh fruit juice increases and improves the blood-content. It is powerful in overcoming *pitta*-aggravation. By adding small amounts of powdered cinnamon and cloves, the stomachic properties of the juice are greatly enhanced.

Ayurvedic as well as Unani systems value this precious plant.

In Profile

Botanical Name	:	*Punica granatun* L.	
English Name	:	Pomegranate.	
Indian Names	:	Assamese	: *Dalim*
		Bengali	: *Dalimb*
		Gujarati	: *Dalamb Dadam*
		Hindi	: *Anar*
		Kannada	: *Dalimbari*
		Kashmiri	: *Daan*
		Malayalam	: *Mathulam Pazham*
		Marathi	: *Dalimb*
		Oriya	: *Dalimba*
		Punjabi	: *Anar*
		Sanskrit	: *Dalima*
		Tamil	: *Mathulam Pazham*
		Telugu	: *Dannima Pandu*
		Urdu	: *Anar*
Family	:	Punicaceae.	
Appearance	:	Glabrous shrub or small tree, with narrowly elliptic or lanceolate leaves; bright red flowers and orange-coloured funnel-shaped calyx tube. Fruit, large globose berry, yellowish red when ripe with persistent calyx lobes. Seeds surrounded by edible, succulent pinkish white pulp.	

Distribution	:	Cultivated throughout India.
Medicinal Parts	:	Stem, stem-bark, root, seeds, buds, flowers, fruit, pulp, juice, rind, seed oil, etc.

In Tradition

AILMENT	PRESCRIPTION
✤ Anaemia	: Dissolve $1/4$ tsp cinnamon and 2 tsp honey in 1 cup pomegranate juice and drink.
✤ Anaemic conditions, burning sensation during urination, sexual debility	: Grind 2 or 3 tsp dried seeds and take once or twice along with milk.
✤ Intestinal worms	: Mix 1 tsp root-bark and 4 to 5 crushed cloves. Make a decoction by boiling in water. Cool and drink. (A purgative is often taken after this treatment.)
✤ Dysentery	: 1 tsp finely powered rind and $1/4$ tsp nutmeg mixed with 1 tsp ghee, taken once or twice a day.
	: Grind 10 pomegranate flowers in $1/2$ cup water. Strain. Take 1 tbsp daily.
✤ Passing of blood along with urine, bleeding piles, blood dysentery	: $1/2$ tsp each powder of dried pomegranate flowers, khuskhus and dried neem leaves, taken twice a day along with milk.

233

❦ Bleeding piles, : 1 tbsp flower juice mixed with sugar
passing of blood candy, taken twice daily.
along with stools,
stomach upset

❦ Infertility : Fine powder of seeds and bark is mixed
in equal quantity. $1/2$ teaspoonful of
this mixture is taken along with hot
water twice a day for a few weeks.

❦ Leucorrhoea : Mix 1 tbsp powder of rind in a mug of
water. Use as a vaginal douche frequently.

❦ Sagging breasts : Heat 4 tsp neem oil and mix 1 tsp
dried and powdered rind. Allow it to
boil for sometime. Cool and use as
massage oil.

❦ Uterine infection : A drink is made by boiling 5–6 flowers
in a cup of water; the filtrate is mixed
with 1 teacup milk and sugar to taste.

❦ Vaginal itching : Powder: 3 tsp saunf, 2 tsp lily-of-the-
valley root, $1/2$ tsp pomegranate flower,
$1/2$ tsp rose-hips. Sift. *Dosage:* 1 to
2 tsp daily with 1 teacup buttermilk or
juice of green grapes.

❦ Asthma, cough : Mix juices of fresh ginger, pomegranate
and honey in equal quantities. Take
1 tbsp of this mixture once or twice a
day.

❦ Boils : Fine powder of dried rind is mixed with
warm mustard oil and applied.

❧ Sores, ulcers,   : Apply a smooth paste of the rind on
haemorrhoids   the affected parts.

❧ Burns and scalds   : Grind pomegranate flowers and apply
                           the paste on affected parts.

❧ Aggravation of   : Mix about 1/4 tsp each powdered
pitta, body heat,   rind, cumin, dried ginger and pepper
nausea   in ghee. Take once or twice a day.

❧ Prevents *pitta*-   : Fruit juice taken frequently.
aggravation, body
heat, dysentery,
nausea, fever,
headache, diabetes

Note: Individual results may vary.

A Word of Caution

Excess intake of pomegranate can cause constipation.

Large doses of rind can cause cramps, vomiting and other unpleasant side effects.

In Science

Chary, M. P. et al. 1984. Screening of Indian plants for their anti-fungal principle. *Pesticides* 18(4):17–18.

Charya, M. A. S. et al. 1979. Laboratory evaluation of some medicinal plant extracts against two pathogenic fungi. *New Bot.* 6, 171.

Chopra, C. L. et al. 1960. *In vitro* anti-bacterial activity of oils from Indian medicinal plants I. *Amer. Pharm. Ass. Sci. Ed.* 49:780–781.

Dhawan, B. N. and P. N. Saxena. 1958. Evaluation of some indigenous drugs for stimulant effect on the rat uterus. A preliminary report. *Indian J. Med. Res.* 46:808. (Peel extract showed spasmogenic effect.)

Dholakia, M. V. et al. 1992. Study of *Dadimadi Ghrat. Jour. Res. Ayur. Sid.* XIII, 3–4:169–173. (The uses of an oil-based preparation of pomegranate.)

George, M. et al. 1947. Investigation on anti biotics II. A search for anti biotic substance in some Indian medicinal plants. *J. Sci. Industr. Res.* 6B(3):42–46. (Antibiotics in pomegranate.)

Gujral, M. L. et al. 1960. Oral contraceptives. Part I. Preliminary observations on the antifertility effect of some indigenous drugs. *Indian J. Med. Res.* 48(1):46–51. (Pomegranate as a contraceptive.)

Majumdar, S. K. and S. K. Bose. 1955. Studies on antifungal antibiotics. Part I. Antifungal microorganisms in Indian fruits and vegetables. *J. Sci. Industr. Res.* 14C(7):126–128.

Masilungan, V. A. et al. 1951. Screening of Philippines medicinal plants used in the treatment of tuberculosis for substances inhibitory to *Myobacterium tuberculosis. Philipp. J. Sci.* 88(2):245–251.

Miranda, D. et al. 1993. *In vitro* action of *Dadima* (*Punica granatum* Linn.) against micro-organisms involved in human gastro-intestinal infection—Isolation and identification of tannins. *Jour. Res. Ayur. Sid.* XIV, 3–4: 154–164. (Tannin content of pomegranate is the active principle.)

Naqvi, B. S. et al. 1985. Screening of Pakistani plants for anti-bacterial activity. *Pak. J. Sci. Industr. Res.* 28(4):269–275.

Naqvi, S. A. H. et al. 1992. Anti-amoebic activity of rind and flowers of *Punica granatum. J. Sciences ISI Repub. Iran* 4(1):1–3.

Panossian, A. G. et al. 1980. Search for substances having prostaglandin-like activity in plants. *Khim. Prir. Soedin.* No 6:825–827.

Pillai, N. R. Anti-diarrhoeal activity of *Punica granatum* in experimental animals. *Intl. J. Pharmacognosy.* 30(3):201–204.

Prakash, A. O. and R. Mathur. 1976. Screening of Indian plants for antifertility activity. *Indian J. Exptl. Biol.* 14(5):623–626.

Rojas Hernandez, N. M. and S. Acosta Duenas. 1980. Antifungal potentials in aqueous extracts from Cuban plants. *Rev. Cubana. Farm.* 14(3):325–328. (Pomegranate shows antitumor activity.)

Rao, R. B. et al. 1982. Analytical profile of certain Ayurvedic drugs used in gastro-intestinal disorders. *Nagarjun* 25(10):224–227. (Pomegranate found useful in diarrhoea and dysentery.)

Sahu, T. R. et al. 1983. Further contributions towards ethnobotany of Madhya Pradesh. Plants used against diarrhoea and dysentery. *Ancient Sci. Life* 2(3): 169–170.

Singh, K. P. and G. N. Chaturvedi. 1981. Herbal treatment of giardiasis. *Sachitra Ayurveda* 34(6):401–404. (Flower buds of pomegranate when in combination with other plants showed excellent response.)

Singhal, K. C. 1983. Anthelmintic activity of *Punica granatum* and *Artemesia silversiana* against experimental infections in mice. *Indian J. Pharmacol.* 15(2):119–122. (Stem and root extracts of pomegranate are useful against tape worm.)

Trivedi, V. B. and S. M. Kazmi. 1979. *Kachnar* and *anar* as antibacterial drugs. *Indian Drugs.* 16, 295. (Flower buds exhibit antibacterial activity against *Bacillus* and other test pathogens.)

Venkataraghavan, S. and T. P. Sundaresan. 1981. Short Note on contraceptives in Ayurveda. *J. Sci. Res. Pl. Med.* 2(1&2):39–42. (Contraceptive use of pomegranate.)

Vishwa Prakash et al. 1980. Anthelmintic activity of *Punica granatum* and *Artemesia silversiana*. *Proc. Indian Pharmacol. Soc.* XII, Ann. Conf. Jaipur. *Indian J. Pharmacol.* 12:62. (Extract of pomegranate prevents eggs from hatching into larvae.)

35

Sandalwood

Santalum album

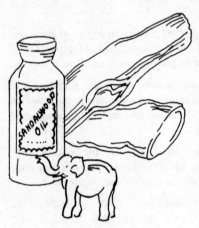

> The endeavours of a man who has studied the entire science but fails to make a clear exposition of the same, are vain like the efforts of an ass that carries a load of sandalwood without ever being able to enjoy its pleasant scent.
>
> —Charaka

The Sadhakas' Aid

Sandalwood has been in use in India right from Vedic times. It was used in a cosmetic ointment called *urguja* along with oil of aloe, rose and jasmine.

Megasthenes, the Greek envoy who came to India in 300 BC, has recorded that the Emperor Chandragupta Maurya used to have an oil massage comprising a mixture of myrrh, aloe and sandalwood.

Like tulsi, sandalwood is considered sacred by the Hindus. It is traditionally believed that sandalwood helps in opening the third eye. Hence it is often applied on the forehead. It is also believed to aid the transmutation of sexual energy into spiritual energy. Meditators or sadhakas use it in the form of agarbathi or as oil or paste or infusion; it is believed that its aroma aids in meditation.

Buddhists and Jains too use sandalwood in their ritual worship. Parsis use its wood for the fire in their temples.

The heartwood of the sandalwood tree is medicinal. It is used externally as a paste or powder to calm skin eruptions. When applied on the skin in the form of a paste, it protects against the sun's radiation. It counteracts wrinkles. It cures inflamed swellings, headache, fevers, hemicrania and other skin eruptions. It helps in allaying inflammation and pruritis.

Internally, sandalwood purifies the blood, cools burning sensations and fevers, and quenches thirst as a weak tea. It however, promotes the production of urine. The alcoholic extract of the stem has experimentally proved its effect on blood pressure.

Sandalwood oil, along with rose oil, is widely used in aroma therapy. It has been experimentally confirmed that the oil possesses anti-microbial activity against fungi. The most important component of sandalwood oil is santalol. Due to its presence, the wood is never attacked by termites and vermin and can last almost indefinitely.

Red sandalwood (*Pterocarpus santalinus*) or *Rakta-Chandana* belongs to a totally different botanical family, but it resembles sandalwood in its properties and action.

The Profile

Botanical Names	:	*Santalum album* L. (Syn. *Sirium myrtifolium* L.)
English Names	:	White Sandalwood, White Saunders, Yellow Sandalwood.
Indian Names	:	Bengali & Gujarati : *Sukhad*

239

Hindi, Marathi & Sanskrit	:	*Chandan*
Tamil	:	*Sandanam*
Telugu	:	*Gandhamu, Srigandapumu*
Urdu	:	*Sandal Safaid*
Family	:	Santalaceae.
Appearance	:	A small tree, which is a root-parasite. It borrows other trees' roots to nourish itself. Flowers, greenish yellow turning brownish purple in cymes. Fruit, black when ripe.
Distribution	:	Common in peninsular India, especially in dry deciduous forests. It has been introduced in Uttar Pradesh, Madhya Pradesh, Rajasthan and Orissa.
Medicinal Parts	:	Heartwood, oil.
Preparation and Dosage	:	*Powder*: 200 mg to 1 g dosage. *Decoction*: Boil 1 heaping tsp wood in 1 cup water. Take 1 to 2 cups a day, a mouthful at a time. *Tincture* : A dose is from 20 to 40 drops.

In Tradition

AILMENT	PRESCRIPTION
❧ Giddiness due to blood pressure	: Soak 1 tsp each powdered amla, coriander seeds and sandalwood in a cup of water overnight. Strain and drink the next day. Continue for a few days.

❧ Diabetes : Mix 1 tsp each sandal paste and amla powder. Boil in a glass of water. Filter and drink.

❧ Pain in heart : Boil $1/2$ tsp sandalwood powder in 1 cup water. Drink thrice daily.

❧ Dysentery : Boil 5 pinches of sandalwood powder in 1 cup water, add a little honey and drink.

❧ Stomach upset : Add 1 tsp sandalwood powder to a cup of water. Add to the resultant emulsion the following: 1 tsp each sugar, honey and the left-over water used to boil rice.

❧ Abdominal pain due to retention of urine : Add $1/2$ tsp camphor and 1 tbsp sandalwood paste to 1 tbsp warm mustard oil. Massage gently over the lower abdomen. (*Note:* This causes the bladder to contract and the urine to flow out.)

❧ Blood in urine (Haematuria) : Soak 1 tsp sandalwood powder in a glass of water overnight. Drink the water next morning. (*Note*: Intake of vegetables like green bananas, bitter gourd and drumstick is recommended.)

❧ Burning sensation during urination : Add 1 to 2 drops of sandalwood oil to milk and take as a night-cap at bedtime.

❧ Fever : Apply sandalwood paste on the forehead to bring the temperature down.

❧ Headache : Grind some tulsi leaves and mix in some sandalwood paste. Apply on the affected areas.

: Mix some coriander seed powder with sandalwood paste and apply on the affected areas.

❧ Gonorrhoea, inflammation of urinary bladder (cystitis), painful urination : Take 5 drops of sandalwood oil along with 1 teacup milk. Add a pinch of powdered ajwain. Drink.

❧ Gonorrhoea, leucoderma, urinogenital infections : Take 1/2 tsp sandalwood powder along with 1 cup milk twice daily. (*Note:* It helps to improve dull complexions.)

❧ Sexual debility : *Panchakalpam* is a Siddha medicine which is prepared by mixing equal quantities of the following five herbal powders: sandalwood, turmeric, chebulic myrobalan, amla and belleric myrobalan. Add a little Malabar Nut leaf juice to bind the powder. Roll it into small tablets. Take 1 tablet every day along with milk for a month.

❧ Acne : Make a paste of 1/2 tsp each sandalwood and turmeric powder in a little water and apply.

❧ Body odour, pimples, skin-allergy

: Mix 1 tsp lime juice with sandalwood paste and apply all over.

❧ Eczema

: Add 1 tsp camphor to 1 tsp sandalwood paste and apply on the affected areas.

❧ Excessive sweating

: Mix dry sandalwood powder in rose water (1:1) and apply over parts where sweating is excessive.

❧ Pimples

: Mix sandalwood oil and mustard oil (1:2). Apply on the affected areas.

: Grind equal quantities of nutmeg, sandalwood and black pepper and apply frequently.

❧ Prickly heat

: Apply sandalwood paste as such or mixed with a paste of neem leaves (1:1).

: Mix 3 tbsp sandalwood powder (dry) and 1 tbsp pure rose water. Apply on the affected areas.

❧ Scars on the face, particularly due to pimples

: Mix equal amounts of sandalwood powder, lime juice and coconut oil and apply on the face before retiring to bed everyday.

❧ Skin-eruptions and lesions

: Apply sandalwood paste on the affected areas.

❧ Pimples, psoriasis, boils, Aids, gonorrhoea

: Boil 1 tsp sandalwood powder in 3 cups water till it is reduced to 1 cup. Add a little rose water and sugar and take thrice a day.

❧ Heat exhaustion   : Apply some sandalwood oil on the forehead.

Note: Individual results may vary.

A Word of Caution

People with high *kapha* or with severe lung congestions should avoid using sandalwood either internally or externally.

In Science

Buchbaner, G. 1977. Sandalwood Oil. *Seifen Fette Wachse.* 103:125. (On sandalwood oil.)

Demole, E. et al. 1976. A chemical investigation of volatile constituents of East Indian sandalwood oil (*Santalum album*). *Helv. Chim. Acta* 159:737. (Chemistry of the volatile oils.)

Dhar, M. L. et al. 1967. Screening of Indian plants for biological activity. Part I. *Indian J. Exp. Biol.* 7:237. (Medicinal properties of sandalwood.)

Frawley, D and V. Lal. 1993. *The Yoga of Herbs.* Delhi: Motilal Banarsi Das. (Sandalwood: an introduction.)

Khanna, Girija. 1994. *All About Herbal Remedies.* Delhi: Tarang Paperbacks. (Folk use of sandalwood and its oil.)

Lust, John. 1974. *The Herb Book.* New York: Bantam Books. (Sandalwood and its use.)

Maruzella, J. C. and P. A. Henry 1958. Anti-microbial activity of perfume oils. *J. Am. Pharm. Ass.* 47:471. (Sandal oil can combat bacteria and germs.)

Nigam, M. C. et al 1983. Status report of Sandalwood oil. *Curr. Res. Med. Arom. Pl.* 1983, 5:124. (On the medicinal applications of sandalwood oil.)

Shankar, R. and R. K. Singhal. 1994. Clinical assessment of the effects of *sandana* (Sandal) *podi*-A in the treatment of *Diabetes mellitus (Neerazhiv)*. *Jour. Res. Ayur. Sid.* XV, 3–4:89–97 (300 mg. administered twice a day for 45 days showed mean fall of sugar-levels, 49.8 mg at fasting and 110.45 mg post-prandial without any side effects or toxic effects.)

Varma, R. R. and N. Vijayamma. 1991. Pharmacological studies on *Rakta Chandana (Pterocarpus santalinus* Linn). *J. Res. Ayur. Sid.* XII, 3–4:190–199. (A decoction of heartwood showed anti-convulsant and anti-inflammatory activities in rats.)

36

Sesame

Sesamum indicum

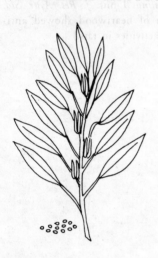

A drop of sesame oil is gently placed with the help of a haystick, on the surface of urine collected in an utensil. If the oil spreads over the surface, the disease is curable. If the oil drop remains suspended, the disease is difficult to cure. If the oil drop setles to the bottom, the disease is incurable.

—Nagarjuna, *'Taila Bindu Pariksha'*, the First Urine Specific Gravity Test.

Treasure of the Living and the Dead

In ancient times sesame was a major source of food, wine and oil and was treated as a royal treasure. It was considered to be a powerful aphrodisiac.

In India, the archaeological recovery of a lump of sesame at Harappa confirms its use by the great civilization of the Indus valley. During the Vedic period, sesame was a sought-after oil-seed for many a ritual, particularly for those connected with death and the dead.

The seeds which possess confirmed medicinal properties vary in colour from yellowish white to black. Once their seed coats are removed, they are cream coloured. They have a pleasant nutty flavour when roasted.

Oil extracted from the seeds, known as gingelly oil, is a popular cooking base. In the traditional cuisine of of South India, it has a key role in imparting its characteristic flavour.

Sesame paste or tahini is a popular and nutritious spread in many countries of the Middle East.

The Profile

Botanical Name	:	*Sesamum indicum* L.
English Names	:	Sesame, Arbenne.
Indian Names	:	Hindi : *Til* Sanskrit : *Tila* Tamil : *Ellu*
Family	:	Pedaliaceae.
Appearance	:	Tall, erect, annual herb. Leaves ovate, grow alternately on the stem and are deeply veined. Flowers whitish yellow. Fruit is a two-celled pod which bursts open when the seeds are ripe. Seeds vary in colour from yellowish white to black.
Distribution	:	Grown mainly in Uttar Pradesh, Madhya Pradesh, Rajasthan, Andhra Pradesh, Maharashtra and Tamil Nadu.
Medicinal Parts	:	Seeds, oil.

In Tradition

AILMENT	PRESCRIPTION
❦ Pain in knee joint or bone joint	: Cut a lime into small pieces. Pack them in a cotton cloth and dip this

bag into hot gingelly oil. Foment the affected joints when bearably hot.

❧ Rheumatic
pains
: Char 2–3 tsp pepper powder in a little gingelly oil. Remove from the fire. When bearably hot, massage the affected areas.

❧ Bedwetting
: Fry 1 tsp crushed coriander seeds in a cast-iron skillet until they are lightly burnt. Mix in 1 tsp each pomegranate flowers, ground sesame seeds and gum acacia. Add brown sugar to equal the amount of powdered herbs. Take 1 tsp at bedtime.

❧ Polyuria (excess
urination in
old age)
: Make a confection of 1 tbsp sesame seeds and 2 tbsp jaggery by mixing them. 1 tsp of this mixture to be taken twice a day for a few days.

❧ Burning
sensation in
eyes
: Mix the juice of bottle gourd and sesame oil (4:1) and heat till the moisture is evaporated completely. Once cool, use it for massaging the head.

❧ Certain types
of deafness,
hearing deficiency
: Cut a colocynth fruit (*Citrullus colocynthus*) into small pieces and fry in 1 teacup gingelly oil till charred. Strain. Put two drops into the ears.

❧ Dandruff
: Grind the leaves into a very fine paste. Apply on the scalp. After 10 mts, rinse.

❧ Earache : Heat 1 tsp garlic in 2 tbsp gingelly oil. Strain. Put 2–3 drops into the ears, when bearably hot.

❧ Pain in ear : Heat 1 tsp each garlic and ajwain in
due to boils, etc 2 tbsp gingelly oil till they turn red in colour. Strain and cool. When cooled to body temperature, put some drops into the ears.

❧ Prevention : Grind the following: Trailing eclipta
of premature (2 parts), black sesame seeds (1 part)
greying and dried amla fruits (1 part). Take 1 tsp with milk and sugar twice daily for a month.

❧ Facial paralysis : A flummery is made by boiling together until a paste like consistency is achieved, 1 teacup each wheat flour, gingelly oil and jaggery to which 1 tsp each cinnamon and dried ginger are added. This is used as a poultice.

❧ Delayed : Add to a glass of milk the following:
menstruation 6–8 crushed almonds, $1/2$ tsp ground sesame powder, 1 tsp honey and an egg yolk. Drink once a day.

❧ Sexual debility : Mix sesame seeds with jaggery and eat.

❧ Phlegm : Heat 1 tsp garlic in 3 tbsp gingelly oil. Rub this preparation on the chest and throat.

❧ Cracks in the feet : Mix the juice of bottle gourd and sesame oil in the ratio 4:1 and heat until all the moisture has evaporated. Bottle and use over cracked skin.

❧ Eczema and other parasitic skin-diseases, ringworm itch, smallpox : Mix a paste of turmeric and neem leaves (1:1) in a little gingelly oil and apply on affected areas.

❧ Kibes : Heat 1 tsp beeswax in 3 tbsp gingelly oil. Add to this 2 tsp finely ground resin. The mixture is further cooked for a few minutes. This ointment is applied when bearably hot on the affected parts.

❧ Whitlow : Take a dhatura fruit and remove the spines. With a sharp spoon, scoop out the pulp. Stuff it with a fine paste of 1 tbsp each turmeric powder and gingelly oil. After stuffing, heat the fruit over a flame. When it is lukewarm, insert the affected finger into it and use it as a bandage. (*Caution:* Dhatura is poisonous.)

❧ Uneven black patches on the face : Make a paste of gingelly oil, milk, turmeric, cumin and black cumin (all equal parts) and apply frequently.

Note: Individual results may vary.

In Science

CSIR. 1972. *The Wealth of India.* Raw Materials. New Delhi. IX. 286.

Library of Tibetan works and Archives. 1994. *Tibetan Medicine.* Series No. 3. Revised Edn. Dharamsala.

Bakhru, H. K. 1992. *Herbs that Heal.* Delhi: Orient Paperbacks.

Dukes, M. N. G. 1980. Remedies used in non-orthodox medicine. *Side Eff. Drugs Annu.* 4:341–347.

Farber, T. M. et al. 1976. The toxicity of brominated sesame oil and brominated soybean oil in miniature swine. *Toxicology* 5:319–335; *Chem. Abstr.* 84:178365.

Kurechi, T. et al. 1980. Transformation of haemoglobin A into metuemoglobin by sesamol. *Life Sci.* 26:1675–1681. (Role of sesamol.)

Lal, S. D. and K. Lata. 1980. Plants used by the Bhat community for regulating fertility. *Econ. Bot.* 34(3):273–275. (Ethno-econo-botanical studies.)

Mupawose, R. M. 1971. Sesame (*Sesamum indicum* Linn.). *Rhod. Agric. J.* 68:121–124,127.

Odebiyi, O. O. and E. A. Sofowar. 1978. Phyto-chemical screening of Nigerian medicinal plants. II. *Lloydia* 41:234–246.

Waray, R. S. 1992. *Shrodhara* and intoxication particularly with reference to withdrawal symptoms. *Deerghayu International.* 8 (4):18–19. (Role of sesame in de-addiction.)

Wilson, R. T. and W. G. Mariam. 1979. Medicinal and magical in central Tigre: a contribution to the ethno-botany of the Ethiopian plateau. *(sic) Econ. Bot.* 33(1):29–34.

37

Cloves

Syzygium aromaticum

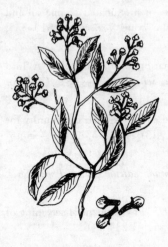

*The Divine Flower, the
Great Flower, the Celestial
Flower...*

—Abhidaana Manjari

The Flower of the Heavens

Clove is one of the most ancient and valuable spices of the Orient.

Charaka Samhita, one of the pioneering works of Ayurveda, describes cloves as the Flower of the Heavens, *Deva Kusuma,* and the Heavenly Aroma as *Divya Gandha.*

Cloves of Commerce

Cloves of commerce come from unopened flower buds which are picked by hand. They are green when picked and acquire a dark brown colour on sun-drying. Unwrinkled brownish-black cloves with a plump and rather rough crown indicate a superior grade.

It is the timing of picking the cloves that determines their quality. If picked early, an inferior product, Khoker cloves, is obtained. If delayed, the flowers get pollinated and fruition occurs.

Cloves in Medicine

Cloves are aromatic, stimulant and carminative and are used in gastric irritation and dyspepsia. They are administered in the form of powder or infusion to relieve nausea or vomiting, to correct flatulence and to invigorate languid digestion.

Steam distillation of clove buds yields a colourless or pale-yellow oil. Clove oil, which darkens with age or exposure, is widely used as a local analgesic for hyper-sensitive dentines and carious cavities. Used externally, it is rubefacient and counter-irritant.

The oil contains a high percentage of eugenol, a naturally occurring anti-oxidant which prevents foods from turning rancid.

Modern medicine eulogises the eugenol in cloves as a drug with incredible medicinal potential. It exerts bactericidal action against *Vibrio cholerae* in a concentration of 1 in 2000. It is also effective against Gartner's bacillus and swine *Erysipelas* bacteria. It inhibits the growth of *Brucella, Mycobacterium, Trichophyton, Achorion* and *Epidermophyton*.

India is an important consumer of cloves and considerable quantities are imported from Tanzania and Singapore.

The Profile

Botanical Name	:	*Syzigium aromaticum* L.
English Names	:	Cloves, Clove Tree

Indian Names	:	Hindi, Bengali, Gujarati,
		Marathi : *Laung*
		Kannada : *Lavanga*
		Malayalam : *Karayampu, Krambu*
		Tamil : *Kirambu*
		Telugu : *Lavangamulu*
Family	:	Myrtaceae.
Appearance	:	A pyramidal or conical evergreen tree about 10 m tall. Bark, smooth, grey. Leaves, lance-like, fragrant, in pairs. Flower buds borne in small clusters at the end of branches, greenish, turning pink at the time of maturity, aromatic. Drupes (mother-of-clove), fleshy, dark pink. Seeds, oblong, soft, grooved on one side.
Distribution	:	Grown in Tamil Nadu (Nilgiris, Courtallam and Kanyakumari) and Kerala (Kottarakkara, Chengannur, valleys of Pamban and Manimala rivers, and in gardens of Pidavoor and Kottayam areas).
Medicinal Parts	:	Dried flower buds (cloves), oil.

In Tradition

AILMENT	PRESCRIPTION
❧ Muscular cramps	: Apply clove oil on the affected parts.
	: Apply clove oil as poultice on the affected areas.
❧ Cholera	: Boil 1 tsp cloves in 10 teacups of water

CLOVES

till it is reduced to 5 teacups. Take in
draughts frequently.

❧ Nausea : Mix powder of fried cloves in 1 teacup
water and drink.

❧ Stomach upset, : Pour 2 to 3 drops of clove oil over
pitta-aggravation sugar candy and eat.

❧ Gum ailments, : Powder of fried cloves (1 tsp) is mixed
throat irritation in 1 teacup lukewarm water and used
for gargling frequently.

❧ Gum and : Apply the powder of fried cloves on
teeth ailments the affected areas.

❧ Headache : Make a smooth paste of cloves, water
and salt. Apply on the affected areas.

❧ Heaviness : Grind 2 to 3 cloves into a fine paste
in head, water along with 1/2 tsp dried ginger
accumulation in and apply on nose, forehead, etc.
head

❧ Toothache : Soak a piece of cotton wool in few
drops of clove oil. Press on affected
areas.

❧ Throat irritation : Chew 2 to 3 cloves with a pinch of
due to coughing common salt.

❧ Nausea in the : Mix 2 tsp powder of fried cloves in
case of pregnant 1 teacup boiling water and allow it to
women, lack of steep for 30 mts. Drink 1 tbsp of
appetite this solution frequently.

255

✦ Bronchial disease : Boil 6 to 8 cloves in 1 tbsp water. A
teaspoon of this decoction is taken with
honey frequently.

Note: Individual results may vary.

A Word of Caution

Cloves, due to their pungency, produce heat in the body. Intake
of cloves is to be avoided in cases of hypertension, high *pitta* and
inflammatory conditions.

In Science

Biswas, S. K. ed. 1957. *R. Ghosh's Pharmacology, Materia Medica and
Therapeutics including Applied Pharmacology.* 20th Edn. Calcutta:
Hilton and Co. (The therapeutic effects of cloves.)

Guenther, E. 1948–1952. *The Essential Oils.* 7 vols. New York: D. Van
Nostrand Co. Inc.

Nayak, K. P. and N. K. Dutta. 1961. Role of Essential Oils and Allied
Drugs in experimental cholera of the rabbit. *Indian J. Med. Res.*
49:51.

Parry, E.G. 1921–22. *The Chemistry of Essential Oils and Artificial
Perfumes.* London: Scott, Greenwood and Sons. (Chemistry of clove
oil.)

Sethi, S. C. and J. S. Agarwal. 1952. Stabilization of Edible Fats by
Spices and Condiments—Part I. *J. Sci. Indutr. Res.* 11B: 468. (Cloves,
when heated with oils and fats, effectively check the development
of rancidity.)

Sethi, S. C. and J. S. Agarwal. 1956. Stabilization of Edible Fats by
Spices—Part II. A New Anti-oxidant from Betel Leaf. *J. Sci. Industr.*

Res. 15B:34. (The anti-oxidant effect of cloves when heated with vegetable oils could be due to the production of stabilizing substances; Iso-eugenol, a major constituent of clove oil exhibits appreciable anti-oxidant effect, when used with vegetable or animal oils.)

Simonsen, J. and W. C. G. Ross. 1947–1957. *The Terpenes Addenda to Vol. V.* Cambridge: Mayo University Press. (Medicinal constituents of clove.)

38

Ajwain

Trachyspermum ammi

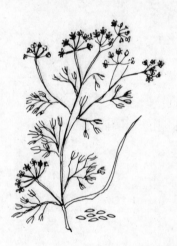

Ajwain alone helps digest a hundred varieties of food.

—An Ancient Sanskrit Saying

The Panacea of All Peoples

Charaka, Sushruta, Galen and Dioscorides all recognized ajwain's immense contribution as a carminative medicine.

Ajwain was traditionally used for the treatment of a number of ailments: dyspepsia, diarrhoea, flatulence, indigestion, spasmodic disorders, microbial infections, etc. It has well-known anti-parasitical properties.

In home medicines, ajwain seeds are used in the form of decoction, aqua or essential oil. They are often used in combination with asafoetida, rock salt, myrobalan, etc.

Recently, when Gujarat was rocked by the suspected cholera

epidemic, there was a mad rush for ajwain. Ajwain water, which is distilled from the seeds (botanically speaking, they are fruits) was administered in the dose of 3 to 4 tbsp to check vomiting in the early stages of this dreadful disease.

There are two varieties of the plant, ajwain: one with long seeds and the other with short ones. It is the short-seeded variety which is preferred for medicinal use.

The Profile

Botanical Names	: *Trachyspermum ammi* L. sprague. *Sison ammi* L. *Carum copticum* Benth & Hook.
English Names	: Bishop's Weed, Ammi, Ajwain.
Indian Names	: Bengali : *Jowan, Joan* Gujarati : *Yavan* Hindi : *Ajwain* Kannada : *Oma* Kashmiri : *Jawind* Malayalam : *Omum* Marathi : *Onva* Oriya : *Juani* Punjabi : *Ajowain* Sanskrit : *Ajamoda Yavanika* Tamil : *Omum* Telugu : *Vamu* Urdu : *Ajowain*
Family	: Umbelliferae.
Appearance	: Small, erect, annual herbs with soft fine hairs. Leaves, feather-like. Fruits are strong-smelling, small, egg-shaped and grey in colour.
Distribution	: Cultivated throughout India.
Medicinal Parts	: Fruits.
Preparation	: Infusion, decoction, medicated oil and powder.

In Tradition

AILMENT   PRESCRIPTION

❧ Loss of appetite   : Mix and powder equal quantities of ajwain, saunf, dried ginger, salt and caraway seeds (*Carum carvi*). Mix a teaspoon of this powder in cooked rice along with ghee and eat frequently.

❧ Flatulence, lack of appetite (also recommended for disorders relating to liver, stomach, intestines)   : Soak 3 tbsp ajwain seeds in an adequate quantity of lime juice and dry in the shade. When fully dried, powder with a little black salt. Take 1 tsp of this mixture twice daily for a few days with a little warm water. (This treatment is more effective when fats and spices are avoided in the diet.)

❧ Colic pains, gas problems, gastralgia, indigestion, repeated belching, pain in the abdomen around the navel   : Grind 2 tsp each ajwain and dried ginger into a fine powder. Add a little black salt. Take 1 tsp of this mixture with 1 teacup warm water frequently. (This treatment is more effective when all types of solid food are avoided for 24 hours.)

❧ Kidney-pain, renal colic   : Mix and grind 1 tbsp black cumin seeds, 2 tsp ajwain seeds and 1 tsp black salt into a fine powder. Add 1 tsp vinegar. Take 1 tsp dose of this mixture every hour till symptoms subside. (*Note*: Do not prolong this treatment for more than a day at a stretch.)

❧ Earache

: Add $1/2$ tsp ajwain seeds to 1 tbsp boiling milk. Cool. Filter. Use as ear drops.

❧ Earache, boils inside the ear, etc

: Heat 2 tsp mustard oil. Add $1/2$ tsp ajwain seeds and one or two flakes of crushed garlic. Boil till they turn red. Filter. Use as ear drops.

❧ Migraine

: Roll some ajwain seeds in a piece of tissue paper. Light it and smoke like a cigarette.

❧ Nasal congestion in children

: Crush a fistful of ajwain seeds and tie up in a cotton napkin and place it near the pillow.

❧ Sexual debility

: Fry equal quantities of ajwain seeds and kernel of tamarind seeds in ghee. Powder and store in a dry, cool place. Mix 1 tsp of this powder in a glass of milk along with 1 tbsp honey. Drink daily at bedtime.

❧ Asthma, bronchial problems, etc

: Roll a fistful of ajwain seeds in cotton cloth. Heat this bundle on a tawa and apply on chest and neck when bearably hot.

❧ Common cold

: Take $1/4$ tsp ajwain powder and 1 tsp turmeric powder in a bowl. Add 1 teacup hot water. Take 1 tbsp with 1 tsp honey.

❧ Common cold, nasal congestion

: Take a pan containing boiling water. Add 1 tbsp crushed ajwain seeds and inhale the vapours frequently.

❖ Common   : Add to ¹/₂ litre of boiling water, 1 tsp
cold, congestion   ajwain seed powder along with 1 tsp
in chest   turmeric powder. Cool. Take 1 tbsp of
                    this mixture along with 1 tsp honey.

❖ Cough   : Mix ¹/₂ tsp ajwain seeds, 2 cloves and
                    a pinch of salt. Powder and sip with a
                    little warm water frequently.

❖ Respiratory   : Crush 2 tsp ajwain seeds. Mix in a
problems due to   glass of buttermilk and drink.
blockage of dried
phlegm

❖ Fainting, giddiness : A hot poultice of seeds used as dry
                    fomentation for hands and feet.

Note: Individual results may vary.

A Word of Caution

Persons prone to hyper-acidity and high *pitta* should avoid
frequent use of ajwain.

Use of ajwain should generally be avoided in summer months
and in very hot climates.

In Science

Atal, C. K. and B. M. Kapur. 1982. *Cultivation and utilisation of aromatic plants.* Jammu-Tawi: Regional Research Laboratory. CSIR.

Central Council for Research in Ayurveda and Siddha. 1990. *Phytochemical Investigations of Certain Medicinal Plants used in Ayurveda.* 231. New Delhi. (Recent phytochemical research on ajwain.)

Chopra, R. N. et al. 1969. *Glossary of Indian Medicinal Plants.* 245. New Delhi: Council of Scientific and Industrial Research, and its *Supplement,* 1969, 97. (Fruits yielded an essential oil containing thymol.)

Dikshit, A. and A. Hussain. 1984. Anti-fungal action of some essential oils against animal pathogens. *Filoterapia* 55(3):171.

Harborne, J. B. and C. A. Williams. 1972. *Phytochemistry* 11, 1741. (Seeds showed the presence of thymol.)

Srivastava, K. C. 1988. Extract of a spice *Omum (Trachyspermum ammi)* has anti-aggregatory effects and alters arachidonic acid metabolism in human platelets. *Prostaglandins Leukotriienes Essent.* 33(1):1; *Chem. Abstr.,* 1988, *109,* 12745 a.

39

Fenugreek
Trigonella foenum-graecum

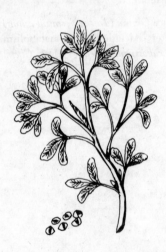

*Methi balances vata,
eliminates fevers...*

—Bhaava Prakasam

The Traveller Who Came to Stay

Historically speaking, the Indian subcontinent has not only offered refuge to different human races hailing from different corners of the world, but also to plants of different hues and uses.

Originating from Eastern Europe, fenugreek, popularly known as methi, has merged with Indian cuisine in such a way that it is well-nigh impossible to make many Indian recipes without it.

Fenugreek grows in abundance in North India, particularly in Gujarat and Maharashtra. Well over 20,000 tonnes of fenugreek are produced in India, of which a sizeable quantity is also exported to other countries.

Medicinally, fenugreek seeds soothe down persistent coughs. Large amounts of the decoction are given to those suffering from tuberculosis or recovering from an illness. It can be taken for fever and bronchitis. It helps in restoring a deadened sense of taste or smell. It can be a useful gargle for sore throats.

The seeds are rich in iron and hence helpful in combating anaemia. They are used externally in poultices for boils, abcesses and ulcers and internally as an emollient for inflammation of the intestinal tract. In the southern parts of India, they are used as a partial substitute for blackgram in the preparation of batter for dosa. It has been analysed that supplementation of raw or germinated seeds at the rate of ten per cent level increases the biological value of the batter.

Both leaves and seeds help in cooling down the body. Hence it can be ideally included in the diet, particularly during the hot summer months.

Steaming is reported to be the best method of cooking the leaves from the point of view of availability of the vitamins and also palatability.

The Profile

Botanical Name	:	*Trigonella foenum-graecum.*
English Name	:	Fenugreek.
Indian Names	:	Bengali, Gujarati, Hindi, Oriya, Marathi, Punjabi, Sanskrit &
		Urdu : *Methi*
		Kannada : *Menthya*
		Malayalam : *Ventayam, Uluva*
		Tamil : *Vendhayam*
		Telugu : *Mentulu*
Chinese Name	:	*Hu Lu Ba.*

Family	:	Leguminoseae.
Appearance	:	Strong-scented, erect, robust, annual herb with light-green, pinnate, tri-foliate leaves. Flowers, yellow. Pods, beaked. Seeds, brownish yellow with peculiar odour; oblong with a deep groove across one corner.
Distribution	:	Cultivated widely in North India, particularly in Maharashtra and Gujarat.
Medicinal Parts	:	Seeds, leaves.
Preparation and Dosage	:	Powder (250 mg to 1 g dosage), paste, gruel, decoction.

In Tradition

AILMENT	PRESCRIPTION
✤ Furuncle, gouty pains, neuralgia, sciatica, skin-irritations, swollen glands, sores, tumours, wounds	: Make a poultice of pulverized seeds.
✤ Pain in hips	: Cook 1 cup leaves together with an egg and 1 cup coconut milk. Eat once a day for 2–3 days.
✤ Anaemia	: 2 tsp fenugreek seeds cooked with 1 cup rice. Eaten with a little salt regularly for a fortnight.

	: Cooked fenugreek leaves eaten regularly.
Angina pectoris	: Boil 1 tsp fenugreek seeds in 1$^1/_2$ cups water. Strain and add 2 tsp honey. Take twice daily.
Diabetes (early stage)	: 2 tsp powdered seeds taken daily with milk (alternatively, this may be soaked in a cup of water at night and the water taken in the early morning and the seeds eaten as such or with honey). The treatment should continue at least for a month.
Hypo-function of liver, indigestion	: Allow the seeds to sprout and eat with breakfast.
Biliousness, stomach problems	: Fenugreek leaves, boiled and fried in butter and eaten twice daily.
Biliousness, giddiness, headache, insomnia	: 2 tsp fresh juice of fenugreek leaves along with 1 tsp honey taken daily.
Constipation, duodenal ulcers, failing eyesight, piles	: Boil 1 cup leaves and eat with honey. Twice daily.
Constipation, cough, mouth ulcer, piles, sore-throat	: Boil 2 tbsp fenugreek leaves along with $^1/_2$ cup moong dal and 10 small onions and eat regularly.
Dysentery	: Soak 2 tsp fenugreek seeds in coconut water or in buttermilk for a few hours. Strain and drink.

	: Fenugreek seeds, fried and powdered, mixed with honey; thrice daily.
❧ Stomach ache, stomach burn	: Take 1 tsp fenugreek seed powder along with milk or buttermilk twice daily for a few days.
❧ Stomach ache, stomach upset, intestinal worms, mouth ulcer	: Methi seeds, fried and powdered. This is added to drinking water. 2–3 times daily for 2–3 days.
❧ Stomach ache, liver problems	: Fenugreek seeds, mustard seeds, asafoetida and turmeric, all in equal quantities, fried in ghee and powdered. This powder (3 to 4 tsp) is mixed with rice and eaten every day for a week.
❧ Pain during urination, stomach ache	: Mix $1/2$ tsp powdered seeds in buttermilk and drink.
❧ Fever, body odour, mouth odour	: Tea made by boiling 1 tsp fenugreek seeds, taken twice or thrice a day. (A little honey or lemon juice can be added to improve the flavour.)
❧ Baldness, falling hair	: Fenugreek seeds, ground in water and applied on the head. Allow to soak at least 40 mts before washing. Every morning for a month.
❧ Burning sensation in eyes, failing eyesight	: Mix equal quantities of fenugreek seed powder along with shikakai powder for washing hair. Wash frequently.

❧ Falling hair, dullness and coarseness of hair	: Fresh leaf paste applied over scalp before bath.
❧ Mouth ulcer, sore throat	: An infusion of leaves gargled 5–6 times daily for a couple of days.
❧ Sexual debility	: Boil 1 cup leaves and mix with 1 tsp each almond and khuskhus. Add wheat flour and ghee and make into paranthas.
❧ To increase lactation in mothers	: Mix $1/2$ tsp powdered seeds along with dalia (cracked wheat) or rice porridge and eat daily.
❧ Sexual debility	: Boil 1 tsp ground seeds in 1 cup water and drink.
❧ Blackheads, wrinkles, pimples	: Fresh leaf paste applied on face every night before going to bed and washed off with warm water next morning.
❧ Boils, swellings	: Leaf paste, heated and when lukewarm, applied on the affected parts of the body.
❧ Boils, ulcers, sores	: Grind seeds into a paste and apply on the affected parts.

Note: Individual results may vary.

A Word of Caution

Pregnant women are advised to avoid fenugreek in their diet as it may cause vaginal bleeding.

In Science

Ahmed, K. et al. 1953. Choline contents of some common Bengal foodstuffs. *Indian J. Med. Res.* 47:563. (Choline content of fenugreek.)

Bhavsar, G. C. et al. 1980. Studies on *Trigonella foenum-graecum* Linn. *Indian J. Pharm. Sci.* 42:39–40.

Chauhan, D.V.S. 1968. *Vegetable Production in India.* Agra: Ram Prasad & Sons. (On the crop and its cultivation.)

Chopra, R. N. et al. 1956. *Glossary of Indian Medicinal Plants.* New Delhi: Council of Scientific and Industrial Research. (Methi's medicinal role.)

Chopra, R. N. et al. 1958. *Indigenous Drugs of India: Their Medical or Economic Aspects.* Calcutta: U.N. Dhur & Sons. (Fenugreek as a component of home remedies.)

Choudhury, B. 1967. *Vegetables.* New Delhi: National Book Trust. (A general account of fenugreek.)

Dixit, B. S. and S. N. Srivastava. 1977. Detection of diosgenin in the seeds of *Trigonella foenum-graecum* Linn. *Indian J. Pharm.* 39:62. (0.38% diosgenin noticed by gas-liquid chromatography method.)

Dixit, B. S. et al. 1985. Analysis of induced mutants of *Trigonella foenum-graecum. J. Econ. Taxon. Bot.* 6:337–340.

Dixit, B. S. et al. 1985. Induced variation in diosgenin content of fenugreek (*Trigonella foenum-graecum L*). *Sachitra Ayurv.* 37:437–439. (Diosgenin production in fenugreek.)

Jain, S. C. and M. Purohit. 1980. Anti-cancerous reagents from some selected Indian medicinal plants I: Screening studies against *Sarcoma ascites, J. Res. Ayur. Sid.* VIII, 1–2:70–73. (Water-extract of fenugreek possessed significant anti-tumour activity.)

Laxmi, V. and S. K. Datta. 1986. Gamma ray induced small seeded mutant of fenugreek. *J. Nucl. Agric. Biol.* 15(3):193–194.

Laxmi, V. and S. K. Datta. 1986. Induction and analysis of MMS induced mutant of fenugreek. Sci & Cult. 52: 310–312. (Effect of radiation.)

Nahar, N. 1993. Medicinal Plants in the treatment of Diabetes. *Traditional Medicine* 205–209. New Delhi: Oxford-IBH. (The test-sample viz. the whole powder and its extracts showed hypoglycemic effects in post-prandial condition. The efficacy increased when the extracts were given simultaneously with glucose load. However, there was no effect in fasting state.)

Pahwa, M. L. 1990. Effect of methi intake on blood sugar in humans. *Oriental J. Chem. 6(2):*124–126. (Anti-diabetic role of fenugreek.)

Pavithran, K. 1994. Fenugreek in *Diabetes mellitus* (letter). *Jour. Assoc. Physicians India* 42(7):584 (Anti-diabetic action of fenugreek.)

Shankaracharya, N. B. and C. P. Natarajan. 1972. Fenugreek—Chemical composition and uses. *Indian Spices* vol IX no 1. p 1–11. (A general survey.)

Singhal, P. C. et al. 1982. Hypocholesterolaemic effect of *Trigonella foenum-graecum* (methi) *Curr. Sci.* 51(3):136–137. (Fenugreek can bring down the cholesterol level.)

Smith, F. and R. Montgomery. 1959. *Chemistry of Plant Gums and Mucilages.* New York: Reinhold Publishing Corporation. (Chemical components of fenugreek.)

Steinmetz, E. F. 1954. *Materia Medica Vegetabilis.* 3 vols. Holland.

Watt, J. M. and M.G. Breyer-Brandwijk. 1962. *The Medicinal and Poisonous Plants of Southern and Eastern Africa.* 2nd edn. Edinburgh. E. & S. Livingstone Ltd.

Whyte, R. O. 1957. *The Grassland and Fodder Resources of India.* Scientific Monograph No. 22. New Delhi: Indian Council of Agricultural Research.

Yagna Narayan Aiyer, A. K. 1958. *Fieldcrops of India with special reference to Mysore.* 5th edition. Bangalore. p 346. (Special reference to fenugreek.)

40

Ginger

Zingiber officinale

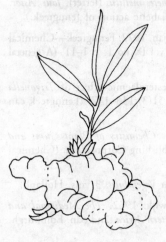

> There's no restriction for
> chukku
> that it could cure only this
> and not that.
>
> —An Agasthyar Song in
> Tamil.

The Oldest Universal Medicine

Ginger, which is referred to as *Vishwa-Bhesaj*, the Universal
Medicine, originates in Indian soil.

India is the largest producer and exporter of this precious
rhizome. Seventy per cent of the produce comes from a single
state: Kerala.

Ginger was highly esteemed by the ancient Greeks and
Romans who obtained it from India through Arabian traders via
the Red Sea. It was introduced into France and Germany in the
9th Century and to England in the 10th Century. It is now
cultivated in several parts of the world.

Ginger promotes digestive power, cleanses the throat and
tongue, dispels cardiac disorders and cures nausea, cough,

anorexia, anaemia, fever, flatulence, constipation, swelling, etc.
It is useful in diarrhoea, cholera, dyspepsia, neurological diseases,
diabetes, eye diseases, etc. It is also prescribed as an adjunct to
many tonic and stimulating remedies.

Both fresh and dried ginger have almost identical medicinal
qualities. However, while some view dried ginger as a better
stimulant and expectorant, fresh ginger is attributed to be a better
diaphoretic, better for cold, cough, nausea and for deranged *pitta*.

The Profile

Botanical Name	:	*Zingiber officinale* Roc.	
English Names	:	Race Ginger, Black Ginger, African Ginger.	
Indian Names	:	Bengali	: *Ada*
		Gujarati	: *Adu*
		Hindi	: *Adrak* (fresh), *Sonth* (dried)
		Kannada	: *Shunti, Ardraka*
		Malayalam	: *Andrakam, Inji*
		Marathi	: *Ale*
		Oriya	: *Ada*
		Punjabi	: *Adrak*
		Sanskrit	: *Ardraka*
		Tamil	: *Inji* (fresh), *Chukku* (dried)
		Telugu	: *Allamu, Sonti* (dried)
		Urdu	: *Adrak, Adhrak*
		Ayurvedic	: *Ardraka*
		Unani	: *Zanjafil*
Chinese Names	:	*Gan Jiang* (dried); *Shen Jiang* (fresh).	
Appearance	:	Erect perennial herb with aromatic rhizome. Stem, erect 15–150 cm tall, covered with leaf sheath. The sterile flowers are white with purple streaks and grow in spikes.	

Distribution	:	Hot, humid areas of South India, Assam and Himachal Pradesh.
Medicinal Parts	:	Rootstock (rhizome).
Preparation and Dosage	:	*Infusion:* Mix 1/2 tsp powdered rootstock with 1 tsp honey. Add 1 cup boiling water.
		Tincture: Take 15 or more drops at a time, warm. If desired, an ounce of brandy or other liquor can also be added.
		Powder: 1/2 tsp in warm water with honey.

In Tradition

AILMENT | PRESCRIPTION

❧ Swelling in hands and feet : Blend 1 teacup each juice of ginger and madar leaf and dhatura leaf. Boil it and cool. Apply on affected parts.

❧ Arthritis : Combine 6 tsp each ginger and caraway seeds along with 3 tsp black pepper into a fine powder and preserve. Take 1/2 tsp with water twice daily.

❧ Backache : First smear ginger paste on the affected area. Over this apply oil of eucalyptus.

❧ Joint pain, rheumatic pain : A 3-inch piece of dried ginger is ground with a grape-sized piece of asafoetida in milk. The paste is applied on the affected area. The area is exposed to the sun for imparting warmth and heat.

❧ Sprain : Add to a hot water bath the following:

274

$1/2$ cup each ginger powder and baking soda and 1 tsp eucalyptus oil.

❧ Dyspepsia, nausea and vomiting due to biliousness, indigestion, jaundice, morning sickness, piles, etc : $1/2$ tsp ginger juice with 1 tsp each fresh lime and pudina juice mixed with a tbsp of honey, taken frequently.

❧ Dysentery : Juice applied around the navel.

❧ Gas problems : Add to 1 cup water a powdered mixture of 1 tsp each cardamom and ginger. Add a pinch of asafoetida and drink.

: Crush some ginger and extract the juice. Dissolve some asafoetida in it. Apply over the stomach.

❧ Indigestion : Grind 1 tsp each saunf, dried ginger and cloves into a fine powder. Add honey to make a thick paste. Preserve. Take 1 tsp 15 mts after each meal and before bedtime.

: Mix 1 tsp rock salt into $1/2$ cup each ginger water and lime juice. Preserve in a glass bottle and expose it to the sun for 3 to 4 days. *Dosage:* Mix 1 tsp with $1/2$ cup water. Take twice daily after meals.

❧ Loss of appetite, stomach ache : 1-inch piece of dried ginger is cut into small pieces and boiled in 2 cups water. After mixing it with milk and sugar, take it frequently like tea.

❦ Nausea and vomiting
: A mixture of juices of ginger and raw onions (1–3 tsp) taken with honey.

❦ Constipation
: Make a fine powder of 1 tsp each ginger (dried or fresh), saunf, senna leaves and rock salt, and preserve. Take 1 tsp with water at bedtime.

❦ Diarrhoea
: Combine 1 tsp each of the powders of ginger, cinnamon and cumin. Add honey to make a thick paste. Take 1/2 to 1 tsp thrice daily.

: Grind 3 tsp ginger and 5 tsp saunf into powder. Add honey to make a thick paste. Take 1 tsp in tea thrice daily and before bedtime.

: Blend together 1 tsp grated (fresh) ginger along with a little nutmeg powder, 1/2 cup water and 1/2 cup yoghurt. Drink.

❦ Fever
: 1 tsp fresh ginger juice mixed with a cup of fenugreek decoction and 1 tsp honey.

❦ Earache
: A few drops of ginger juice used as ear drops.

❦ Gum inflammation
: Mix 1/2 tsp salt with 1 cup ginger water. Apply by dipping finger in water and rubbing on gums.

❧ Headache   : Rub dry ginger with a little water on a grinding stone and apply on the forehead or affected areas.

                                  : Apply ginger paste (after heating) slightly on affected areas. (*Note:* Ignore the initial burning sensations.)

                                  : Apply a paste of $1/2$ tsp ginger powder mixed with water and heated.

❧ Toothache   : Paste of dry ginger applied to gums along with a little salt.

❧ Sore throat   : Chew a small piece of fresh ginger.

❧ Painful, irregular   : A piece of fresh ginger, ground and
   menstruation   boiled in a cup of water. The infusion is taken thrice daily after meals along with sugar.

❧ Sexual debility   : $1/2$ tsp ginger juice mixed with honey and a semi-boiled egg, taken at night.

❧ Asthma   : Pour $1 1/2$ cups hot water over 1 tsp ground ginger. Take 1 tsp lukewarm at bedtime.

❧ Asthma, cough,   : A mixture of juices of ginger and
   etc   pomegranate mixed with honey, all in equal quantity. Take 1 tbsp frequently.

❧ Bronchial asthma   : Powder of equal quantities of dried ginger, pepper and long pepper, taken thrice daily (it can be mixed with honey or can be added to tea). 1 tsp dosage.

❧ Cold

: Ginger pieces, boiled in a glass of water and taken after straining with $1/2$ tsp sugar.

❧ Common cold

: Boil in 2 teacups water, 1 tbsp grated fresh ginger, 1 tsp cinnamon powder and 1 tsp liquorice. Take 1 cup of this decoction once every 3 hours, sweetened by 1 tsp honey.

: Boil 1 tbsp fresh ginger paste, 1 tsp each liquorice and cinnamon powder in 1 cup water for 10 mts. Add honey and drink.

❧ Cough

: Prepare a tea of $1/2$ tsp each ginger paste, cloves and cinnamon powder. Add honey and drink.

: Juice of ginger taken with honey 2–3 times daily.

❧ Sinus

: Inhale the steam from a tea of ginger or eucalyptus leaves.

❧ Whooping cough

: A mixture of juices of ginger, lemon and onions, all in equal quantities in 1 tbsp dosage, taken frequently.

❧ Boils

: Apply a paste of ginger powder and turmeric (1:1) on boils.

❧ Facial wrinkles, premature greying, senility

: Soak shredded ginger in honey. Eat a spoonful every morning.

❧ Old age problems : Boil 1 tsp ginger in 1 cup water till reduced to $1/2$ cup. Add to it $1/2$ cup cow's milk, 2 pieces of cardamom, 5 strands of saffron and 1 tsp granulated sugar. Drink every morning.

❧ To wean away : Boil some ginger in 1 cup water till
from intoxicants it is reduced to $1/2$ cup. Add $1/2$ cup
and drugs cow's milk, 2 cardamoms and 1 tsp honey, and drink every day.

Note: Individual results may vary.

Ginger Pill

Mix fresh ginger juice along with dried ginger powder (4:1 ratio) with the help of a mortar and pestle, until the mixture takes on a jam-like consistency. Roll into pea-size pills and store. Take one pill thrice a day.

Ginger Tonic

Mix thinly sliced ginger with cardamoms, honey, saffron, and rose petals. Keep in a glass jar under the sun. Take 1 tsp of this tonic every day for forty days. Avoid meat, tobacco, coffee, tea and spices.

Ginger Jam

After removing the rind, slice the ginger (a big piece) into fine julienne strips. Add $1/4$ tsp cardamom seeds, 3 tbsp honey, a few pinches of saffron and a few rose petals.

Keep this inside a glass jar and under the sun. Remove and

store. Take 1 tsp in the morning for 40 days. (Avoid meat, spices, tobacco, coffee and tea for best results.) Useful in cases of stomach upset, indigestion, weakness of heart, body heat, phlegm-accumulation, etc.

A Word of Caution

Patients suffering from high fever, bleeding, ulcers, inflammatory skin diseases, etc may avoid the use of ginger. The constitution of the patient needs to be taken into account before prescribing ginger.

The outer rind of both fresh as well as dried ginger needs to be discarded before use.

Ginger relieves *kapha* when taken along with honey; *pitta* when consumed with rock candy; *vata,* with rock salt.

In Science

Denyer, C. V. et al. 1994. Isolation of anti-rhino viral sesquiterpenes from ginger (*Zingiber officinale*). *J. Nat. Prod.* 57(5):620–628. (Chemistry of the anti-viral principle.)

Kawai, T. et al. 1990. Anti-emetic principles of *Magnolia ovata* bark and *Zingiber officinale* rhizome. *Planta Med.* 0(1):17–20. (How ginger stops vomiting.)

Lee, C. Y. et al. 1982. Study on the anti-oxidative activities of spices grown in Taiwan. *Chung-kuo Nung Yeh Hua Hsues Hui Chih* 20(1–2):61; *Chem. Abstr.* 1982, 97, 143288p. (Anti-oxidative activities of ginger.)

Mathai, C. K. 1975. Seasonal accumulation of chemical constituents in ginger varieties (*Zingiber officinale* Roscoe.) *J. Plantation Crops.* 3(2): 61–64.

Mitsubhishi Chemical Industries. 1980. Gingerols as cardio-tonic agents. *Jpn. Kokai Tokyo Koho JP.* 8259; *Chem. Abstr.* 1982, 97, 33378k.

Sethi, S. C. and J. S. Agarwal. 1952. Stabilization of Edible Fats by Spices and Condiments. Part I. *J. Sci. Industr. Res.* 11B:46. (Dried ginger effectively checks the development of rancidity in vegetable oils.)

Shoji, N. et al. 1982. Cardiotonic principles of ginger. *J. Pharmo. Sci.* 71(10):1174. (Effective principles in ginger.)

Suekawa, M. et al. 1984. Pharmacological studies on Ginger I. Pharmacological actions of pungent constituents, (6)—gingerol and 6—shogaol. *J. Pharmacobio-Dyn.* 7 (11) 836; *Chem. Abstr.* 102, 72421k.

Glossary of English Medical Terms

Abortifacient: Causing abortion.

Abscess: Local inflammation of body tissues with deep suppuration caused by bacteria which destroy the cells in the centre of the area and leave a cavity filled with pus.

Acidity: Excess of hydrochloric acid found in the stomach.

Acne: Skin condition, found usually in adolescents, in which glands of skin get infected.

Adaptogenic: Anti-stress.

Adenoma: Tumour consisting of glandular material.

Adenopathy: Glandular disease.

Adrenal: Located near the kidneys.

Alkaloids: Nitrogenous compounds in plants, sometimes the most powerful poisons.

Alopecia: Baldness.

Allergy: Abnormal sensitivity to any substance.

Amenorrhoea: Delayed menstruation.

Amoebic infection: Infection caused by amoeba, a single-celled protozoan.

Amphetamine: Powerful synthetic drug which stimulates the heart and respiration, constricts blood vessels and induces sleeplessness.

Anaemia: A decrease in the volume of blood or some of the normal constituents of blood, causing paleness.

Analgesic: Relieving pain.

Androgen: Any organic compound which promotes development of masculine characteristics.

Anaesthetic: A substance which produces loss of some form of sensitivity or entire loss of sensibility.

Angina pectoris: Severe pain over the heart.

Anodyne: A medicine that allays pain.

Anorexia: Loss of appetite, marked, or extreme.

Anthrax: Disease of man from animals; two forms exist, one of the skin and the other of the lungs.

Antibiotics: Extracts from the lower plants (eg. moulds) which are used to cure a number of infectious diseases. If the higher plants are not used in the manufacture of antibiotics, it must be remembered that their growth is very slow in comparison with moulds and other lower plants.

Anticoagulant: Reducing the clotting tendencies of blood.

Antidote: Remedy given to counteract a poison.

Antiemetic: Preventing vomiting.

Antihypertensive: Lowering blood pressure.

Antioxidant: A substance capable of delaying or preventing rancidity or deterioration of quality in food.

Antipyretic: Reducing fever.

Antiseptic: Inhibiting growth of, or destroying germs.

Antispasmodic: Relieving or preventing spasms.

Anti-tussive: Relieving coughing.

Aphrodisiac: An agent or drug which excites sexual activity.

Appetite-loss: Aversion to food.

Arteriosclerosis: Hardening of arteries.

Artery: A member of that portion of the circulatory system which conveys blood away from the heart.

Arthritis: An abnormal accumulation of fluid in the peritoneal cavity.

Ascites: (also *Dropsy*) An accumulation of body fluids in the abdomen.

Ascorbic Acid: Vitamin C, occurring in fresh fruits.

Asthmatic problems: Periodic attacks of difficulty in breathing.

Astringent: Firming tissues and organs; reducing secretions.

Atony: A condition of muscular relaxation characterized by complete absence of postural contraction.

Atrophy: Wasting of a tissue or an organ.

Backache: Pain in the spine or its adjacent areas.

Baldness: Lack of hair.

Bacterium (pl. Bacteria): Single-celled organisms which bring about decay, disease or build up nitrogen compounds in the soil.

Bactericidal: Destroying bacteria.

Bedsores: Lesions over pressure areas on the body of a bedridden patient.

*Bedwetting (*also, *Nocturia):* Frequent urination at night.

GLOSSARY OF ENGLISH MEDICAL TERMS

Bile: The external secretion of the liver; a brownish or yellowish fluid of bitter taste, which aids digestion both by producing an alkaline reaction in the small intestine and by promoting the emulsification and absorption of fat, and which acts as a vehicle for the elimination of a variety of excretory products.

Biliousness: Mild upset of the liver caused by dietary indiscretion.

Bitter Principles: A group of substances having a common property, i.e. the bitter taste having therapeutic significance, although their constituents may belong to different and unrelated chemical groups.

Bladder: Collecting pouch for urine from kidneys.

Bleeding: Emitting blood. Bleeding can result from a small cut or wound and will usually clot of its own accord.

Blood: Fluid contained in arteries and veins of the body that carries nutrients to and waste away from all tissues. Made up of cells and plasma.

Blood pressure, Low: See Hypotension.

Blood pressure, High: See Hypertension.

Brachycardia: An abnormally slow rate of heart-beat.

Bronchitis: An inflammation of the mucous lining of the bronchial tubes.

Carbuncle: Large boil; an infection of skin and subcutaneous tissue by *Staphylococcus aureus.*

Carcinogen: Cancer-producing substance or agent.

Carcinoma: Cancer, especially of epithelial origin.

Cardiac: Of the heart.

Cardiotonic: Tonic for the heart.

Carminative: Expelling gas from the stomach and intestines.

Cataract: Any opacity of the crystalline lens of the eye.

Cathertic: Purgative.

Chest: Area enclosed by the ribs and sternum.

Chest congestion: Accumulation of mucus in chest.

Chest diseases: Respiratory diseases.

Chickenpox: Mild eruptive disease with some resemblance to smallpox, chiefly affecting children.

Cholera: Epidemic disease with violent vomiting and purging, cramps and collapse, endemic in India and epidemic elsewhere.

Cholesterol: Steroid alcohol present in animal cells and body fluids.

Chronic: A term applied to certain disorders, denoting their slow onset and persistant duration.

Cirrhosis: Over-growth of an organ.

CNS: Central Nervous System.

Coagulant: Coagulating agent.

Cold: Inflammatory condition of mucous membrane of nose and throat, with catarrh.

Colic: Acute abdominal griping pain caused by various abnormal conditions in the bowels.

Colitis: Inflammation of the colon.

Colon: The longest portion of the large intestine.

Congestion: An abnormal accumulation of blood or lymph in some organ or region of the body.

Conjunctivitis: Inflammation of the transparent membrane covering the eyeball.

Constipation: Condition of bowels in which defaecation is irregular and difficult.

Contraceptive: Preventive of uterine conception.

Contusions: Bruises.

Convulsion: A violent contraction of an extensive group of muscles, brought about by the action of the Central Nervous System.

Corns: Horny induration of cuticle with hard centre and root, sometimes penetrating deep into the subjacent tissues, caused by undue pressure, chiefly of boots or shoes on feet.

Cortisone: A harmone produced by the adrenal glands.

Cough: Sudden expiratory movement produced by irritation of the larynx, trachea, bronchi, or pleura.

Counter-irritant: Thing used to produce surface irritation and thus counteract symptoms of disease.

Cracks: Fissures formed by breakage.

Cramp: A violent contraction of some group or groups of muscles maintained for a considerable period without relaxation.

Cystitis: Inflammation of the bladder.

Dandruff: Condition of the scalp characterized by dry scaling.

Deafness: Complete or partial loss of hearing.

Dehydration: Loss of water.

Debility: Abnormal lack of force or vigour in the vital functions.

Delirium: A state of more or less clouding of consciousness, dream-like incoherent notions, illusions, and hallucinations, and restlessness or stupor, most common with fever or on a toxic pasis, usually with poor memory of the experience.

Demulcent: A drug which exerts a local soothing action, especially on the mucous membrane.

Depression: A feeling of melancholy, hopelessness and dejection.

Diabetes: Disease characterized by excessive discharge of glucose-containing urine, with thirst and emaciation, caused by the failure of pancreas to secrete an adequate amount of insulin and the resultant accumulation of glucose in the blood.

Diagnosis: Identification of disease by investigation of symptoms and history.

Diaphoretic: Producing or increasing perspiration.

Diarrhoea: Excessive looseness of bowels.

Digestion: The motor and chemical process by which nutritive substances are ingested, carried along the alimentary tract, and rendered capable of absorption into the blood and lymph.

Diphtheria: Disease causing the development of membrane in nose and throat.

Distension: Act of stretching.

Diuretic: An agent which increases the formation of urine.

Dizziness: Any sensation of imbalance in the interaction with immediate environment.

Dropsy: Generalized accumulation of fluid in body; edema.

Dysentery: Disease with inflammation of mucous membrane and glands of large intestine and mucous and bloody evacuations.

Dysfunction: Impairment of function.

Dyspepsia: Indigestion or impaired digestion.

Dyspnea: Laboured breathing.

Earache: Pain in ear, usually due to inflammation.

Eczema: An itching disease of the skin.

Ejaculation: Ejection of semen.

Ejaculation, involuntary: See Nocturnal emission.

Emetic: Producing vomiting.

Elephantiasis: Tropical disease in which blocking of the lymph vessels by a parasite leads to great swelling of the tissues, especially in the lower limbs.

Emmenagogue: Stimulating or restoring menstrual flow.

Emollient: Softening and soothing.

Enteritis: Inflammation of the intestinal tract by infection or irritating food.

Epilepsy: A nervous disorder, usually chronic, with characteristic convulsions of sudden onset, a tonic spasm often with crying and arrest of breathing followed by twitching, biting of tongue, frothing at the mouth, relaxation of the sphincter.

Epiphora: Continuous overflow of tears.

Erysipelas: Infection of the skin with *streptococci.*

Exhaustion: The limiting case of muscular fatigue, in which the stimulus or excitation ceases to elicit any overt motor response whatever.

Expectorant: Causing or stimulating expectoration to cough up and spit.

Fainting: Temporary loss of consciousness due to insufficient blood reaching the brain.

Fatigue: Exhaustion.

Fever: Elevation of body temperature.

Febrifuge: Eliminating fever.

Flatulence: Wind or gas in the stomach or intestines.

Flavonoids: A group of glycosides, colourless or pale yellow in colour, which strengthen the blood capillaries and sometimes relieve cramps of the smooth muscles.

Flu (also, *Influenza*): Virus infection characterized by fever, inflammation of the nose, larynx and bronchi, neuralgic and muscular pains and gastrointestinal disorder.

Freckles: Small patches of pigmented skin, more commonly found in people with fair complexion.

Fungal infection: Infection of fungus.

Fungus: Mould.

Furuncle: Boil.

Galactagogue: Increasing milk-secretion.

Gall Bladder: Sac beneath the liver which stores bile and secretes mucus.

Gallstones: Stone-like objects composed mainly of calcium, found in gall bladder and its drainage system.

Gangrene: Death and deterioration of a part of body, caused by interference with the blood supply.

Gastric: Of the stomach.

Gastric secretion: Digestive secretion inside the stomach.

Gastritis: Inflammation of the stomach.

Giddiness: See Dizziness.

Glaucoma: A disease characterized by abnormally high pressure of the fluids within the eye ball, with consequent pain and impairment or loss of vision.

Glycosides: Most active toxic substance found in plants, sometimes used medicinally (eg. fox-glove). Flavonoids and Saponins constitute distinguishable groups of glycosides, which are medicinally useful.

Goitre: Enlargement of the thyroid gland.

Gonorrhoea: An inflammatory disease of the urino-genital passage characterized by pain or discharge.

Glossary of English Medical Terms

Gout: A disease of the purine metabolism, characterized by attacks of arthritis with an associated, raised serum uric acid.

Gums: The tissues and membranes surrounding the teeth.

Gynaecology: Study of the diseases of women.

Gynaecological disorders: Disorders and diseases relating to women.

Haematuria: The passing of blood in the urine.

Haemoglobin: Red-coloured oxygen carrier in RBC.

Haemophilia: Strong tendency to bleed.

Haemoptysis: Spitting up of blood from the lungs.

Haemorrhage: Severe loss of blood from a blood vessel.

Haemostatic: Stopping the bleeding.

Halitosis: Offensive odour of the breath.

Headache: Pain or ache localized in the head.

Helmintic: Expelling or destroying worms.

Hemicrania: Headache confined to one side.

Hemiplegia: Partial paralysis.

Hepatic: A drug that acts on the liver.

Hepatitis: A swelling and soreness of the liver.

Hiccup, hiccough: Spasmodic contraction of the diaphragm causing inspiration, followed by closure of the glottis.

Histamine: Substance naturally present in the body, responsible for complex, physiological phenomena, especially in connection with the work of blood vessels.

Hydrophobia: Aversion to water, especially as symptom of rabies in man; rabies in man.

Hypertension: High arterial pressure.

Hypotension: Low blood pressure; a fall in blood pressure below the normal range.

Hypotensive: Lowering blood pressure.

Hypoglycaemia: Abnormally low level of blood sugar.

Hysteria: A psychoneurosis, resulting from a conflict between the ego and the primitive tendencies of the id, in which the latter tendencies are repressed, and are thus excluded from the direct conscious expression, it being assumed that the unconscious, repressed material finds an indirect physical outlet through conversion, producing the hysterical symptoms.

Immunization: Protection of an organism through inoculation, against specific germs or disease.

288

Immunology: Study of immunity from diseases.

Injury: Any damage inflicted upon an organism. An impairment of structure function, not due to the ordinary biological processes.

Insomnia: Chronic inability to sleep.

Insulin: The active product of the internal secretion of the Islands or Islets of Langerhans in the pancreas.

Intestinal parasites: Bacteria, etc that are parasitical and harbour in the intestine.

Intestinal problems: Disorders in the intestine.

Intestinal worms: Worms that are parasitical, found in the intestine.

Intestine: The membranous tube which extends from the stomach to the anus.

Ischaemia: A local, usually temporary deficiency of blood.

Itch (also *itching*): An irritating cutaneous and internal disorder; a sensory experience which involves mild pricking-pain sensations, unpleasantness, and a persistent impulse to scratch.

Jaundice: Increase in bile-pigments in blood.

Kibe: Ulcerated chilblain, especially on heel.

Kidneys: The vital organs of the human body, which remove waste products from the blood and regulate the amount of water and the delicate balance of chemicals in the body.

Knee: The point of junction of the femur and tibia.

Larva: First stage of an insect from the egg.

Larvicides: Agent which kills larvae.

Laxative: Promoting bowel movements.

Leprosy: Chronic endemic bacterial disease caused by *Mycobacterium lepriae.* Characterized by thickening and ulceration of the skin with loss of sensation and in severe cases deformity and blindness.

Latex: Milky substances found in some plants.

Leucoderma: Depigmentation of the skin.

Leucorrhoea: An abnormal mucus discharge from the vagina.

Leukaemia: A fatal disease of the organs that manufacture blood, such as the lymph glands and bone marrow.

Louse (*pl. Lice*): A wingless blood-sucking insect, *Pediculus humanus,* infests man and acts as the agent in transmiting many diseases.

Lumbago: Back ache in the loin region.

Lymph: Special functioning fluid that flows through specific vessels, passing through the filtre of the lymph glands before entering the blood stream.

Malaria: Acute, febrile, infectious disease caused by the presence of parasitic organisms in the red blood cells.

Glossary of English Medical Terms

Malignant: Cancerous.

Measles: An infectious viral disease marked by fever, a rash of pink spots, redness of the eyes and mild bronchitis.

Melancholia: Depression and self-pity.

Melanin: Black or dark-brown pigment, which imparts colour to the skin.

Memory: Recall of past experience.

Menorrhagia: Excessively profuse menstrual discharge.

Metabolism: Energy exchanges in a living organism.

Migraine: A pathological headache, often on only one side, characterized by nausea and sensory disturbances.

Morning sickness: Nausea and vomiting during the early stages of pregnancy.

Mucilage: In plants, it has the property of swelling in water to produce plastic masses or viscous solutions and hence can be used as a laxative and for the protection of the inflamed mucosa of the digestive tract.

Mucus: A thick, white liquid secreted by mucous glands.

Mumps: An acute infectious disease caused by a virus.

Muscle: The tissue which is responsible for body movement.

Myocardial infarction: Death of a part of the heart muscle. It is caused by a reduction or complete stoppage of the blood supply in the area of the heart.

Myocardial necrosis: See Myocardial infarction.

Myopia: A refractive defect of certain eyes, such that, with relaxed accommodation of the lens, parallel rays of light are brought to a focus before they reach the retina.

Narcotic: A drug which induces narcosis, a condition of stupor, diminished sensitivity to pain, motor paralysis and a tendency towards sleep.

Nausea: A complex sensation of varying genesis and unpleasant affective tone, accompanied by a tendency to gastric contraction and by vomiting.

Neck: Part of the body connecting the head and the trunk.

Necrosis: Death of a part of the body due to absence of blood supply.

Nephritis: Inflammation of the kidneys.

Neuralgia: A painful disorder of one or more nerves. It usually causes sharp, fitful pains.

Nervine: Strengthening the nervous system; may be stimulants and sedatives.

Nervous disease, Nervous disorder: A kind of disorder of the nervous system and its function.

Nervous system: The totality of neurons in the body of any organism.

290

Neuralgia: A nervous disorder characterized by sharp intermittent pain, usually limited to a single nerve, and due to nutritive or functional conditions in the nerve or nerves concerned.

Neurasthenia: A condition characterized by lack of physical and mental vigour, by abnormal fatiguability, and often by the presence of phobias.

Neuritis: An inflamed condition of a peripheral nerve, accompanied by pain and other disturbances both of sensation and of motion.

Nocturnal emissions: The involuntary ejaculation of semen during sleep.

Obesity: A bodily condition in which there is an excess of fat in relation to other bodily components. The condition is presumed to exist when an individual is twenty per cent or more over the normal weight.

Oedema: A swelling, an abnormal accumulation of fluid in cells.

Ophthalmia: An inflammation of the superficial tissue of the eye, especially of the conjunctiva.

Osteo: (*Prefix*) Bone.

Orchitis: Inflammation affecting the testis and characterized by hypertrophy, pain and a sensation of weight.

Osteoporosis: A disorder that causes a gradual decrease in both the amount and strength of bone tissues.

Oxytocin: Hormone produced by pituitary gland, stimulating muscle of uterus.

Oxytocic: Stimulating contraction of the uterine muscle and thus speeding up child-birth.

Pain: A specific sensation stimulated by powerful processes in various bodily tissues, the impulse being commonly assumed to be conveyed by a distinct set of nerves having a ready motor outlet.

Pancreas: Gland lying behind and below the stomach which produces ferments which are passed into the intestinal tract to help in digestion; site of insulin production.

Paralysis: Impairment or complete loss of motor function due to some disturbance of the neural or muscular mechanism; impairment or destruction of sensory function.

Paraplegia: A stroke on one side, particularly the lower section of the body.

Pathogenic: Capable of producing disease.

Pathogens: Anything capable of producing disease.

Penis: Male sex organ.

Peptic ulcer: A non-cancerous crater-like sore in the wall of the stomach or intestine.

Peritonitis: Inflammation of the lining tissue of the abdominal cavity.

Pharmaceutical: Of the use or sale of medicinal drugs.

291

Pharmacology: The study of drugs.

Pharmacy: Preparation and dispensing of drugs.

Pharmacopoeia: Book containing list of drugs with directions for use.

Pharynx: Membraneous tube extending from oral cavity to first part of oesophagus.

Pharyngitis: Inflammation of the pharynx.

Phlegm: Thick mucus from respiratory tract.

Piles: Enlarged painful veins in rectum or around anus.

Pimple: Small pointed area on skin, at times filled with infectious material.

Pituitary gland: A small compound endocrine gland, situated at the base of the brain.

Plague: Epidemic disease, transmitted by fleas or rats. There are two major types: bubonic (which causes swollen lymph glands) and pneumonic (which attacks lungs).

Platelet: Small disc in blood stream, used for blood coagulation.

Pneumonia: A general disease in which the essential lesion is an inflammation of the spongy tissue of the lung with consolidation of the alveolar exudate.

Polio (also *Poliomyelitis, Infantile Paralysis):* A disease that causes paralysis.

Polyuria: Excessive urination.

Poultice: A soft mush prepared by various substances with oily or watery fluids.

Pox: Blisters and scars on the skin caused by certain diseases.

Prickly heat: Irritation of the skin in which blisters form due to increased temperature.

Proctitis: Inflammation of the rectum or anus.

Prophylactic effect: Guarding against; pertaining to the prevention of the development of a disease.

Prostate: Large gland, accessory to male generative organs and surrounding neck of bladder and commencement of urethra.

Pruritis: Itching.

Psoriasis: Chronic skin disease in which red scaly patches develop.

Pulmonary: Of, in, connected with lungs.

Purgative: Drug to relieve constipation.

Pustules: Pimples.

Pyorrhea: Infection of the gums which causes the edges of the tooth sockets to bleed easily when teeth are being brushed.

RBC: Red Blood Corpuscle.

Regeneration: The restoration or replacement of an injured or lost part of the body; renewal of vigour or vitality.

Rejuvenation: The process of restoring vitality, especially the renewal of youthful physiological vigour in a senescent organism.

Renal: Located in the kidneys.

Reproduction: Begetting offspring.

Reproductive: Pertaining to reproduction.

Resins: They are non-volatile secretions; they are used as skin irritants.

Respiration: Breathing.

Respiratory: Pertaining to respiration.

Restorative: Having the power to restore or renew health.

Rheumatism: Pain, swelling and deformity of joints of unknown cause.

Ringworm: Fungus infection.

Roundworm: An intestinal parasite.

Rubefacient: Causing redness, as of the skin.

Saliva: Fluid secreted by the glands of the mouth.

Salivation: Excess secretion of saliva.

Saponins: A group of Glycosides, useful as detergents. Large doses of them in the blood-stream may prove fatal due to haemolysis (by dissolving the red blood corpuscles). Since they are feebly absorbed from the gastro-intestinal tract, their oral administration is generally without danger. They are mild laxatives, diuretics and expectorants.

Scabies: Contagious skin disease due to a parasite, the mite *Sarcoptis scabiei.*

Scald: Burn of skin; the lesion caused by contact with a hot liquid or vapour.

Scalds due to burns: The lesions caused by burns.

Sciatica: Inflammation of or injury to the sciatic nerve in back of thigh.

Sclerosis: Hardening of tissues.

Scrofula: Tuberculous gland of the neck.

Sedation: Treatment by sedatives.

Sedative: Tending to soothe.

Semen: Male secretion containing sperm.

Senility: Old age.

Serum: Amber-coloured liquid which separates from clot, when blood coagulates.

Sexual: Pertaining to sex.

Sinus: A cavity, diverticulum or sac in an organism.

Sinusitis: Inflammation of the nasal sinuses.

Skin: Outer covering of body.

Sleeplessness: Lack of sleep.

Sneezing: A nose irritation which causes sudden expulsion of air from mouth and nose.

Sore: An ulcer or wound.

Spasm: Involuntary, sudden and violent muscular contraction, convulsion.

Spasmodic: Causing intermittent spasms.

Speech: Thought expressed in words.

Sperm: Male fertilizing cell.

Spermatogenesis: Developing spermatozoa.

Spinal cord: A cord-like structure consisting mainly of neurons and tracts of neurons situated within the spine or back bone.

Spleen: A ductless gland, situated at the left side of the cardiac end of the stomach.

Splenitis: Inflammation of the spleen.

Spleen enlargement: See Splenitis.

Sprain: Injury of a joint caused by over-stretching of the ligament.

Sterility: Inability to reproduce; inability to have children.

Stimulant: Increasing internal heat and strengthening metabolism and circulation.

Stomach: A sac-like enlargement of the ailmentary tract, following the esophagus, in which the preliminary process of digestion takes place.

Stomach ache (also *Stomachalgia*): Pain in the stomach.

Stomachic: Strengthening stomach functions.

Stool: Faeces.

Stress: Pressure of load, weight, some adverse force or influence, etc.

Suppurating wounds: Wounds having pus.

Sweat: Perspiration.

Swellings: Inflammation.

Syphilis: Veneral disease caused by *Treponema pallidum.*

TB (also *Tuberculosis*): Infectious disease of man and animals, caused by tubercle bacilli, having many and varied manifestations in lungs, brain, bone, etc.

Tachycardia: Excessive rapidity in the action of the heart.

Tannins: Widespread in plants, particularly in bark, leaves, etc. They aid in healing, as they prevent bacterial growth. They contract blood-capillaries and so prevent certain haemorrhages.

Tape worm: Type of intestinal worm.

Taste: Sensation through nerves on tongue.

Tastelessness: Loss of taste.

Testicles: The male reproductive glands.

Teratology: (Biol.) Study of monstrosities or abnormal formations, especially in man.

Therapeutic: That which treats medically; curative.

Thirst: Desire for liquid.

Thread worm: Parasitic worm.

Throat: Area between mouth and oesophagus.

Tinea: Ringworm.

Thyroid: Located below the larynx.

Tonic: Strengthening organs or the entire organism.

Toxin: Poisonous substance of animal or vegetable origin.

Toxic: Poisonous.

Toxicity of plants: Some plants contain fatal poisons. Because an active constituent is of natural origin, it does not mean that it is non-toxic; obviously both the active constituent and the plant itself may turn out to be poisonous.

Toxicology: Study of the nature and effects of poisons, their detection and treatment.

Tumour: A swelling or growth.

Typhoid: An infectious fever caused by the typhoid bacillus, characterized by diarrhoea and other symptoms.

Ulcer: Sores on skin or internal parts of body, caused by various factors.

Ulcerative colitis: An inflamed condition of the colon and rectum, which are the lowermost portions of the bowel.

Urethra: The duct by which urine is discharged from the bladder.

Urinary bladder inflammation: Inflamation of the bladder.

Urinary problems: Problems pertaining to urine and urination.

Urinary infection: Infection in urinary tract.

Urine: The excretion of the kidneys, stored in the bladder and discharged through the urethra.

Urticaria: Nettle-rash.

Uterus: Womb, a sac-like structure, present in mammals, in which the embryo develops.

Vagina: The passage connecting the outer and inner female sex organs.

Vaginitis: Inflammation of vagina.

Vasoconstrictor: An agent that narrows the blood vessels, thus raising blood pressure.

Vasodilator: Causing relaxation of the blood vessels, thus lowering the blood pressure.

295

Vein: A duct which conveys blood towards the heart.

Venereal disease: Pertains to infectious diseases which may be transmitted by coitus.

Ventricle: One of the chambers of the heart.

Vermicidal: Killing worms in the intestines.

Vermifuge: Substance that expels worms from intestines.

Vertebra: One of the series of bones or cartilages which form the vertebral or spinal column.

Vertigo: Dizziness.

Viruses: Minute organisms that cause diseases such as common cold, measles, mumps, poliomyelitis, chickenpox, smallpox, etc.

Viral infection: Infection caused by viruses.

Vitiligo: Lack of pigment in certain areas of the skin.

Vomiting: The forcible expulsion of substance from the stomach through the mouth, elicited by intestinal, gastric, cardiac, or pharyngeal irritation.

Wart: A circumscribed cutaneous excrescence.

Wound: An injury or break in the skin.

Wrinkle: Furrow-like crease, depression or ridge in skin.

Whitlow: Infected finger.

Glossary of Non-English Terms

Agni: biological fire governing metabolism; cosmic force of transformation.

Ama: toxins; undigested food or uneliminated waste materials.

Ayurveda: the knowledge (*veda*) concerning the maintenance of life (*ayus*), as taught in Atharva Veda.

Bhavaprakasa: a 16th-century text on Indian medicines.

Bhutas: spirits; elements.

Charaka Samhita: a treatise exposition of Ayurveda, compiled by Charaka, with a conceptual framework and approach very much akin to contemporary medicine.

Churan: (also, *Churanam, Churna*) powder.

Dasmool: (also *Dasamoolam*) (the Ten Roots) An Ayurvedic preparation containing a mixture of ten roots, (Bel *Aegle marmelos*, Malay bushbeech *Gmelina arborea*, Agnimantha *Premna serratifolia*, Patala *Stereospermum tetragonum*, Sonapatha *Oroxylum indicum*, Indian Nightshade *Solanum indicum*, the white-fruited variety of the same plant, Shalaparni *Desmodium gangeticum*, Prshniparni *Pseudarthria viscida* and Gokhru *Tribulus terrestris*), which is mainly used to control *vata* anywhere in the body in such varied conditions as asthma, colic, toothache, etc.

Dhatus: the seven basic tissue-elements of the body; the products of digestion.

Dosha: the three essential factors or 'humours' that govern all the biological processes of the living organism are referred to as *doshas* or *tridoshas*; the determinants of individual constitution. The three *doshas* are: *vata, pitta* and *kapha.*

Gulkand: a confection made of petals, usually of rose petals.

Guna: quality; attribute.

Kapha (also *Sleshma*): the bodily water humour; it implies the functions of heat-regulation and also formation of various preservative fluids, e.g., mucus, synovia, etc.

Kayakalpa: a treatment that arrests or retards the ageing process.

GLOSSARY OF NON-ENGLISH TERMS

Kari: a South Indian dish of fried greens or vegetables.

Krimi: a parasitic worm; micro-organisms and other sources of infection.

Kuberā: the Hindu god of wealth.

Lakshmi: the Hindu goddess of wealth, beauty, grace and prosperity.

Lavana: salt.

Leha (also *Leham*): a medicinal jam, prepared by cooking the herbal powder or paste in milk or water to which ghee, sugar syrup, etc are added.

Mantra: special seed-syllables that transmit cosmic energy.

Medhya: a drug which is capable of improving intellect and memory-power.

Nasya: administration of medicines through the nose.

Panchakarma: five types of purification or detoxification conducted on a patient's body.

Pankhuri: the dried petals.

Pitta: the bodily fire humour; it is the manifestation of *tejas* (energy) in the living organism that helps thermogenic and metabolic processes such as digestion, assimilation, tissue building, endocrine activities; etc. *Pitta* in excess causes conditions of anger, acidity, increased body heat, burning sensations, yellowness of body, diminished sleep and excessive hunger and thirst. Insufficient *pitta* causes lack of vigour and joy, coldness, loss of lustre and weakened digestion.

Prana: life-force having five functional variations: *prana, vyana, samana, udana* and *apana.*

Pranayama: breathing exercises that help in mind-control and eventually, relaxation.

Puja: devotional worship usually in elaborate ritual forms.

Purana: the ancient treatises of India which cover roughly the period between the ages of the Vedas and classical literature. The ones of importance in medicine are: *Agni Purana, Brahma Purana, Brahmavaivarta Purana, Kurma Purana, Matsya Purana, Padma Purana, Vamana Purana, Vayu Purana,* etc.

Purusha: primal spirit; principle of sentience.

Rajas, Rajasic: the *guna* linked to activity.

Rakta: blood.

Rasa: initial taste of a substance; essence.

Rasam: a popular South Indian soup, thin in consistency, make of lentils, tamarind, cumin and other ingredients.

Rasayana: a rejuvenative therapy which regenerates body and mind, prevents decay, postpones ageing.

Samana: prana that governs digestive system.

Sambar: a popular soup of South Indian cuisine, somewhat thicker that *rasam,* made of lentils, tamarind, coriander seeds, asafoetida, red chillies and other spices.

Samhita: a section of Vedic literature, generally containing the sacred code of Hindu laws entitled *Smriti*; there are eighteen important samhitas.

Saraswati: the Hindu goddess of learning.

Sattva, Sattvic: principle of light, perception, intelligence and harmony; one of the three *gunas*.

Shakti: the Divine Energy; cosmic feminine principle.

Shiva: the Divine Being; cosmic masculine principle.

Siddha (also, tamil *Siddha*): a yogi from the Tamil country who has attained *siddhi*, super natural powers through intense practices of meditation; a revolutionary and non-conformist in his beliefs and practices; a system of medicine, somewhat akin to *ayurveda*, prevalent in the southern parts of India.

Sloka: a verse.

Soma: the essence energy of the mind and nervous system.

Sraddha: respectful and well-wishing offering to the manes—an obligatory socio-religious rite of the Hindus.

Srotas: bodily channels through which nutrients or wastes move.

Sukla-dhatu: reproductive tissues.

Sukta: epigram.

Susruta Samhita: a treatise compiled by Susruta, similar to *Charaka Samhita*, but with special emphasis on surgery. Susruta described *shalya* or surgery as the highest in value among the therapies because of its ability to produce instantaneous relief by means of instruments and appliances. Sushruta emphasizes that the 'hand of the surgeon is the most important of all instruments.'

Tailam (also *Taila*): medicated oil.

Tamas: tamasic principle of inertia, dullness, darkness and resistance; one of the three *gunas*.

Tantra: a system of the religious worship of the Hindus.

Tridosha: see *Dosha*.

Trikatu: (the Three Pungents) a simple preparation made of ginger, black pepper and long pepper, used to control conditions in which *kapha* or *ama* obstructs *vata*, especially in the respiratory tract.

Triphala: powder of the three myrobalans: emblic or amla, chebulic and belleric.

Udana: *prana* that governs speech, energy, will, memory and exhalation.

Unani: conventional Arabian system of medicine.

Urguja: a cosmetic ointment, prepared from rose, aloe, jasmine, etc.

Vaid, Vaidya: one who is trained in medical science.

Vagabhatta: the author of the treatise *Ashtanga-Hrdaya* (600 A.D.)

Vajikarna: substances that improve sexual vitality and functioning.

Vastu Shastra: This sub veda, also known as *Shilpa Shastra,* on building and town planning is ascribed to Bhrigu, Vasishta, Vishwamitra, Atri and many others. The principal texts are the *Mastsya Purana, Brihad Samhita,* etc.

Vata: (also *Vayu*) the bodily air humour; it explains all the biological phenomena which are controlled by the central and autonomous nervous systems.

Vattal Kuzhamubu: a South Indian soup made of tamarind and dried fruits, somewhat bitter in taste, having medicinal value.

Vedas: ancient scriptures of India, four in number: *Rig, Yajur, Sama* and *Atharva.*

Virya: the energy of a substance as heating or cooling.

Viswa-Bhesaj: a universal medicine, administered to cure very many ailments, hence the name.

Vyana: prana that governs the circulatory system and movement of joints and muscles.

Yantra: mystic diagrams; geometrical designs that manifest cosmic law and channel cosmic energy, drawn on paper or engraved in metal. As an object of worship it takes the place of the image of a particular deity.

Yoga: a methodology of the practical and coordinated application of knowledge; science of self-realization.

Glossary of Plants and Other Ingredients

This glossary covers only those plants which are not discussed under a separate chapter in this book. Abbreviations used: (H)=Hindi; (T)=Tamil.

Aniseeds: *Pimpinella anisum.* A herb with seed-like fruits yielding anise oil, which is used in medicine.

Babchi seeds: *Psoralea corylifolia.* Babchi (H), Kaarbhogam (T). The seeds are traditionally used in the treatment of dermatitis, leucoderma, leprosy, scabies, ulcers, etc.

Ballon vine: *Cardiospermum helicacabum.* Jyotishmati (H), Mudakkaththaan (T). Roots, leaves and seeds of this plant possess medicinal properties. While seeds are tonic, leaves are useful in arthritis. The plant has sedative action on the Central Nervous System.

Betel leaf: *Piper betle.* Paan (H), Vettilai (T). The plant is useful in alcoholism, cough, fever, halitosis, impotency, leprosy, rheumatism, etc.

Bitter orange, Sour orange, Seville orange: *Citrus aurantium* var. *bigardia.* Khatta (H), Naraththai (T). Fruits are useful in vitiated conditions of *pitta* and *kapha,* anaemia, bronchitis, flatulence, nausea, scabies, etc.

Black nightshade: *Solanum nigrum.* Makoy (H), Manathakkaali (T). The plant is useful in vitiated conditions of *tridosha,* asthma, cough, dyspepsia, rheumatalgia, swellings, vomiting, etc.

Bottlegourd: *Lagenaria siceraria.* Lauki (H), Sorakkai (T). The fruits are useful in vitiated conditions of *pitta,* burning of the feet, bronchitis, cough, fainting, fever, inflammation, leprosy, skin diseases, etc.

Bulbils of *Ficus religiosa* (Peepul): Receptacles occurring in pairs and turning purplish when ripe. The dried receptacles, pulverized and taken in water, are reported to cure asthma.

Calamus: *Acorus calamus:* Vacha (H), Vasambu (T). A marshy, aromatic herb, its rootstock, strong-smelling, acid and *pitta,* is known for its memory- enhancing capacity and reduces *vata* and *kapha* but increases *pitta.*

Camphor: *Cinnamomum camphora.* Kapoor (H), Karpooram (T). Camphor is formed in the oil-cells distributed all over the tree, but extracted mainly from the leaves and also from the stems by distillation. It is useful for local application on sprains, inflammations and rheumatic pains. It is also given internally in certain types of diarrhoea or as a cardiac stimulant. It is also useful in vitiated conditions of *vata*, asthma, cough, diarrhoea, flatulence, etc. Camphor is also obtained from another plant, *Ocimum kilimandscharum.*

Caraway seeds: *Carum carvi.* Shahjira (H). The plant is a much-branched herb with leaves finely divided into narrow, lance-shaped lobes, white flowers, strong-smelling seedlike fruits. They balance aggravation of *kapha* and *vata.*

Catechu: The gummy extract of the wood of the Cutch tree, *Acacia catechu.* Katthaa (H), Kaasu-katti (T). It is useful in vitiated conditions of *kapha* and *vata*, anorexia, erysipelas, flatulence, leucoderma, leprosy, skin diseases, ulcers, wounds, etc.

Chicory: *Cichorium intybus.* Kaasni (H), Chikkari (T). An erect, glandular, perennial, milky herb. The plant is useful in anorexia, colic, dyspepsia, flatulence, gout, insomnia, jaundice, skin allergies, etc.

Chitraka: *Plumbago zeylanica.*

Colocynth: *Citrullus colocynthis.* Badi Indraayan (H), Pei-Tummatti (T). An annual herb with leaves deeply divided. Its roots are useful in ascites, jaundice and ophthalmia. Its fruits are useful in asthma, bronchitis, leucoderma, tumour, etc.

Cucumber: *Cucumis sativus.* Khira (H), Vellari (T). A hairy climber with simple leaves. Its fruits are useful in vitiated conditions of *pitta*, burning sensation, fever, general debility, insomnia, jaundice, etc.

Dates: *Phoenix dactylifera.* Khajoor (H), Payreecham (T). A tall palm with pinnate leaves. Its fruits are useful in bronchitis, burning sensation, cough, etc.

Dill: *Anethum graveolens.* Soya (H), Sadakuppi (T). A glabrous, aromatic herb with yellow flowers. Its fruits are useful in asthma, cough, dyspepsia, fever, flatulence, halitosis, inflammation, intestinal worms, syphilis, ulcers, etc.

Dried ginger: Dried rhizomes of *Zingiber officinale.* Sonth (H), Chukku (T).

Drumstick: *Moringa pterygosperma* or *Moringa oleifera.* Sahijan (H), Murungai (T). A graceful tree with grey bark, white flowers and long slender fruits. Its fruits are useful in inflammation, intermittent fever, neuralgia, etc.

Five-leaved chaste tree: *Vitex negundo.* Nirgandi (H), Nalla Nochi (T). An aromatic shrub with quadrangular branches, bluish purple flowers in panicles and globose fruits. Roots, leaves and bark of this plant are used in traditional medicine.

Foxglove: Folk's glove, *Digitalis lanata.* A softly hairy herb with rosette leaves and tall flower spike. Flowers bell-shaped, pink to purple. It is the original source of the heart drug, digitalin.

Gel of aloe: The sap or leaf juice, obtained from *Aloe vera.* The gel is useful in abdominal tumours, amenorrhoea, burns, constipation, flatulence, lumbago, sciatica, etc. *See* also *Indian Aloe*.

Gingelly oil: Oil obtained from seeds of sesame. Til-ka-tel (H), Nallennei (T).

Grapes: *Vitis vinifeara*. Daakh (H), Draakshai (T). A large climber with toothed palm-like leaves with bluish black, purplish, green or yellow fruits. Fruits have medicinal use.

Gular, *See Udumbara*.

Gum: The exudate from plants; widely used in traditional medicine. Resin.

Gum acacia: Gum collected from the branches of *Acacia senegal*.

Gum arabic: *See Indian gum arabic*.

Gum Myrrh: Gum-resin exudate from wounds in the stem of the plant *Commiphora myrrha*, pale-yellow at first, later solidifying into brown-black, collected in Saudi Arabia, Abyssinia, Iran, Thailand and sold in Indian bazaars. This gum is useful in vitiated conditions of *tridosha*. *See* Myrrh.

Henna: *Lawsonia inermis*. Mehendi (H), Marudaani (T). A glabrous shrub with simple leaves, white or rose-coloured fragrant flowers. Its leaves, flowers, roots and seeds are used in traditional medicine.

Horsegram: *Dolichos biflorus*. Kultthi (H), Kollu (T).

Indian acalypha: *Acalypha indica*. Kuppikhokli (H), Kuppaimeni (T). A herb with many branches and egg-shaped leaves and small fruits. Leaves and roots of this plant are useful in bronchitis, constipation, skin diseases and ulcers.

Indian aloe: *Aloe vera* or *Aloe barbadensis*. Ghikumari (H), Kattaalai (T). A coarse perennial with short stem and shallow root system. It has fleshy leaves in rosettes, armed with thorny margins, but decked with yellowish orange flowers. *See Gel of aloe*.

Indian gum arabic: *Acacia nilotica*. Babul (H), Karuvel (T). Gum arabic, which is an exudate from the cuts on the bark, has several medicinal uses. Its colour varies from pale yellow to black.

Indian hemp: *Cannabis sativa*. Bhang (H), Ganja (T). A large, aromatic, resinous herb with palm-like leaves. Although intoxicating, the leaves are medicinally useful in abdominal disorders, convulsions, diarrhoea, etc.

Indian wormwood: *Artemisia nilagirica* or *Artemisia vugaris*. Davana (H), Maasipatri (T). A tall hairy shrub with dissected leaves which are useful in vitiated condition of *kapha* and *vata*, asthma, bronchitis, cough, inflammation, leprosy, skin diseases, etc.

Jamun or Jambu: *Syzigium cumini*. Jamun (H), Naaval (T). A tree with grey bark, having dark patches and simple leaves, greenish white flowers and dark purple fruits with pinkish pulp. Leaves, fruits and bark of this tree have medicinal application.

Kachnar: *Bauhinia variegata.* Kaanchnaar (H), Sigappu Mandarai (T). A tree with vertically cracked grey bark, leaves of two leaflets, white or pink flowers and with long, flat pods. Roots and bark of this plant possess medicinal properties.

Lavender: *Lavendula vera.* A small shrub; native of southern Europe, now grown in Jammu and Kashmir. The flowers are the source of an essential oil, which is used in perfumery.

Latex: A milky fluid present in many plants, mostly white in colour, sometimes yellow or reddish; it consists of a mixture of substances, proteins, gums, carbohydrates, etc.

Lettuce: *Lactuca sativa.* Native of southern Europe and West Asia. Cultivated throughout India. The leaves are eaten as a vegetable.

Linseed or flax-seed: *Linum usitatissimum.* Alsi (H) Alivirai (T). A small herb with lance-like leaves and white-to-blue flowers. Fruits 5-celled capsules. For cattle and horses.

Ma-huang: *Ephedra gerardiana.* Khanda (H). A small herb, found in the drier regions of the temperate and Alpine Himalayas from Kashmir to Sikkim.

Madar: *Calotropis procera.* Madar (H), Vellerekku (T). A common pale grey shrub, with a white cottony fuzz. It is purgative, laxative, abortifacient, aphrodisiac and useful in the treatment of migraine.

Malabar Nut: *Adhatoda vasica.* Vaicka (H), Aadathodai (T). Native to India, it is a common wild evergreen, large-leaved shrub with white or purple flowers. Associated usually with the respiratory system, it is effective as an expectorant and as a cure for asthma. All parts of the plant find medicinal use.

Mastic herb: *Pistacia lentiscus.*

Mould: Fungus.

Myrrh: *Commiphora myrrha.* Bol (H), Vellai Paapolam (T). The gum-resin exudate from wounds in the stem of *Commiphora myrrha,* pale yellow at first, later solidifying into brown-black in colour. *See Gum Myrrh.*

Nendran: a variety of banana available in South India, particularly in Kerala.

Nirbisi: *Cissampelos pareira.* Nirbisi (H), Appatta (T). A wild climber with a long rhizome, kidney-shaped leaves and yellow flowers. Recent laboratory findings indicate fall of blood pressure, respiratory depression, etc, when the drug is administered to animals.

Nux Vomica: *Strychnos nux-vomica.*

Olive: *Olea europea.*

Orange: *Citrus reticulata.* Santara (H), Kamala orange (T). A common tree bearing the most popular fruit.

Palm sugar or Palmyrah sugar: Sugar obtained from the palm, *Borassurs flabellifer.*

Peepul: The tree, *Ficus religiosa.*

Pista: *Pistacia vera.* Pista (H), Pista (T).

Plaksa: *Ficus lacor.*

Prickly chaff-flower: *Achyranthes aspera.* Chiribata (H), Naayuruvi (T). Found in wastelands, it is an erect hairy shrub with barbed fruiting spikes that stick to clothes. Useful in skin and heart ailments and in removing poisons from the body.

Prickly sida: *Sida acuta.* Bariara (H), Mayir Maanickam (T).

Pumpkin: *Cucrbita pepo.*

Quinine bark: *Cinchona officinalis.* Kunain (H), Koina (T).

Radish: *Raphanus sativus.* Muli (H), Mullangi (T). A herb with a white edible tuberous root, yellow flowers and cylindrical pods. Seeds are useful in cough, dyspepsia, flatulence, paralysis, etc.

Rectified alcohol: Alcohol, purified by redistillation.

Red clay: A soft, plastic clay consisting mostly of insoluble substances which have settled down from the surface waters; these substances are partly of volcanic, partly of cosmic origin, and include nodules of manganese and phosphorous, crystals of zeolites, etc.

Resin: The product from the secretion of the sap of certain plants. Resins are hard, fusible, and more or less brittle, insoluble in water, soluble in certain organic solvents.

Sal: *Shorea robusta.* Sal (H), Vellai Kungiliyam (T).

Sage: *Saliva officinalis.* Sej (H).

Senna or Indian senna: *Cassia angustifolia.*

Seasame oil. *See* gingelly oil.

Shikakai: powder: *Acacia concinna* or *Acacia sinuata.* Shikakai (H), Seekkaai (T). A prickly climber with brown branches. Leaves armed with sharp prickles. Flowers, small, globose. Fruits (pods) flat, useful in vitiated conditions of *pitta,* burning sensation, constipation, leprosy, etc.

Slaked lime: Calcium hydroxide, produced when caustic lime is mixed with water, evolving much heat. Chuna (H) Chunaaneku (T).

Sugandha Vacha: *Alpinia officinarum.*

Tailed pepper: Cubebs, *Piper cubeba.* Kabaabchini (H), Vaal-Milagu (T). A climber with ash-grey stems and branches, rooted at the joints, and with simple leaves and small flowers. The dried unripe fruits possess medicinal properties.

Tamarind: *Tamarindus indica.* Imli (H), Puli (T). A large tree with dark grey bark, pinnate leaves, yellow flowers and brownish ash-coloured pods. Its roots, seeds, leaves and fruits find their application in traditional medicine.

Trailing eclipta: *Eclipta alba.* Bhaamgraa (H), Kayyanthagarai (T). A much-branched herb with rooted nodes. Flowers, white, in heads. The plant is reported to be good for blackening and strengthening of the hair.

Triphala: A combination of powders of the Three Myrobalans: amla or emblic (*Phyllanthus emblica*), Chebulic (*Terminalia chebula*) and Belleric (*Terminalia bellirica*).

Bone setter: *Cissus quadrangularis*. Hadjod (H), Pirandai (T). A climber with quadrangular stems, small greenish flowers and red berries. Powdered roots as well as the stem-paste are specific for bone-fracture.

Valerian: *Valeriana officinalis*.

Vetiver: *Vetiveria zizanioides*. Khaskhas (H), Vetbiver (T). A dense perennial grass with aromatic roots and linear, narrow leaves. The roots are useful in anaemia, dyspepsia, flatulence, nausea, skin diseases, ulcers, etc. (Not to be confused with poppy seeds, Khuskhus.)

Violet or Sweet violet. *Viola odorata*.

Wild Emblic: *Phyllantus niruri*. Jungli Amli (H), Keezhaanelli (T). It is a wild, trailing herb. The plant is traditionally used to cure jaundice and liver-diseases.

Wild turmeric: *Curcuma aromatica*. Jungli Haldi (H), Kasturi Manjal (T).

Wormwood: *Artemisia absinthium*.

Yellow-berried nightshade: *Solanum xanthocarpum*. Kantakari (H), Kandankathiri (T). A prickly, bright green shrub, woody at the base with yellowish white prickles. Leaves also armed with prickles. Flowers blue or bluish purple. Fruits yellow or white. Seeds many. The plant is useful in vitiated conditions of *kapha* and *vata,* anorexia, asthma, bronchitis, cardiac disorders, constipation, cough, dyspepsia, epilepsy, fever, flatulence, inflammation, leprosy, lumbago, skin diseases, etc.

Index

Baldness
    Dhatura for, 105–6
    Fenugreek for, 268
    Liquorice for, 138
    Mango for, 150
    Mustard for, 39
Baldness, not due to hereditary factors
    Lime for, 64
    Liquorice for, 137
    Saffron for, 84
Banana, 174–82
Bari Saunf, see Saunf
Barsan, see Curry leaf
Barsanga, see Curry leaf
Basango, see Curry leaf
Bed sores, Banana for, 178
Bed wetting
    Coriander for, 79
    Sesame for, 248
Bel, 2–8
Belching, Ajwain for, 260
Bellulli, see Garlic
Bengal Quince, *see* Bel
Bergeria koenigii, see Curry leaf
Bevu, see Neem
Bhaava Prakaasam, 127
Bhisagarya, 162
Bhursunga, see Curry leaf
Bil Patre, see Bel
Bili, see Bel
Biliousness
    Fenugreek for, 267
    Neem for, 29
    Pudina for, 156
Biliousness, vomiting
    Curry leaf for, 170
    Ginger for, 275
Bilva, see Bel
Bird Pepper, *see* Chilli
Bisharhari, see Curry leaf

Bishop's weed, *see* Ajwain
Bitter Gourd, 161–7
Black Cumin, 191–5
Black dots, Lime for, 66
Black Ginger, *see* Ginger
Black heads, pimples
    Cinnamon for, 58
    Coriander for, 78–9
Black heads, wrinkles, Fenugreek for, 269
Black Mustard, *see* Mustard
Black patches on face, Sesame for, 250
Black Pepper, see Pepper
Bladder stones, Fig for, 123
Bleeding, Liquorice for, 139
Bleeding gums, Pepper for, 221
Bleeding in nose due to body heat
    Coriander for, 78
    Lime for, 64
Bleeding, internal
    Saffron for, 83
    Turmeric for, 96
Bleeding piles
    Bitter Gourd for, 163
    Mango for, 150
    Neem for, 29
    Pomegranate for, 233–4
Blemishes, Lime for, 66
Blond hair, Lime for, 64
Blood deficiency
    Amla for, 214
    Banana for, 177
    Fig for, 123
Blood dysentery, Pomegranate for, 233
Blood impurities, Garlic for, 19
Blood in stools, Pomegranate for, 234
Blood in Urine
    Pomegranate for, 233
    Sandalwood for, 241
Blood infection, Garlic for, 19

INDEX

314

Tongue, loss of taste sensitivity,
   Cinnamon for, 57
Toothache
   Almond for, 227
   Asafoetida for, 119
   Cloves for, 255
   Coconut for, 72
   Ginger for, 277
   Lime for, 65
   Mango for, 149
   Nutmeg for, 187
   Onion for, 12
   Pepper for, 221
Tooth ailments, Cloves for, 255
Tooth, looseness, Neem for, 30
Tooth problems
   Cardamom for, 112–3
   Mango for, 151
   Pudina for, 157
Tooth, yellow
   Almond for, 227
   Lime for, 65
Toxic Fever, Tulsi for, 199
Toxin due to animal bite, Black
   Cumin for, 194
Trachyspermum ammi, see Ajwain
Trigonella foenum-graecum, see
   Fenugreek
Triphala, 211
Trittavu, see Tulsi
Tropical eosinophilia, Garlic for, 20
Tropical skin disease, Turmeric for, 97
Tuberculosis
   Amla for, 215
   Banana for, 178–9
   Bel for, 6
   Garlic for, 20
   Tulsi for, 199
Tuberculosis fever, Tulsi for, 199
Tulasi, see Tulsi

Tulshi, see Tulsi
Tulsi, 196–204
Tumours
   Fenugreek for, 266
   Fig for, 124
Turmeric, 93–102
Typhoid
   Banana for, 179
   Coriander for, 77

Ulcer
   Bel for, 4–5
   Fenugreek for, 267–9
   Neem for, 31
   Pomegranate for, 235
Ulcer, duodenal, Fenugreek for, 267
Ulcer, intestinal, Banana for, 177
Ulcer, mouth
   Amla for, 213
   Bel for, 5
   Coriander for, 78
   Fenugreek for, 267–9
   Fig for, 123–4
   Lime for, 64
   Liquorice for, 138
Ulcer, peptic, Liquorice for, 136–7
Ulcer, stomach, Bel for, 5
Ulcer, uterus, Fig for, 124
Ullipoondu, see Garlic
Uluva, see Fenugreek
Ummam, see Dhatura
Ummattam, see Dhatura
Unconsciousness due to giddiness,
   Onion for, 13
Unpleasant body odour, Tulsi for, 200
Unwanted hair, Turmeric for, 98
Urinary bladder inflammation,
   Sandalwood for, 242
Urinary diseases
   Banana for, 177

READ MORE IN PENGUIN

In every corner of the world, on every subject under the sun, Penguin represents quality and variety—the very best in publishing today.

For complete information about books available from Penguin—including Puffins, Penguin Classics and Arkana—and how to order them, write to us at the appropriate address below. Please note that for copyright reasons the selection of books varies from country to country.

In India: Please write to *Penguin Books India Pvt. Ltd. 11 Community Centre, Panchsheel Park, New Delhi 110017*

In the United Kingdom: Please write to *Dept JC, Penguin Books Ltd. Bath Road, Harmondsworth, West Drayton, Middlesex, UB7 ODA. UK*

In the United States: Please write to *Penguin Putnam Inc., 375 Hudson Street, New York, NY 10014*

In Canada: Please write to *Penguin Books Canada Ltd. 10 Alcorn Avenue, Suite 300, Toronto, Ontario M4V 3B2*

In Australia: Please write to *Penguin Books Australia Ltd. 487, Maroondah Highway, Ring Wood, Victoria 3134*

In New Zealand: Please write to *Penguin Books (NZ) Ltd. Private Bag, Takapuna, Auckland 9*

In the Netherlands: Please write to *Penguin Books Netherlands B.V., Keizersgracht 231 NL-1016 DV Amsterdom*

In Germany : Please write to *Penguin Books Deutschland GmbH, Metzlerstrasse 26, 60595 Frankfurt am Main, Germany*

In Spain: Please write to *Penguin Books S.A., Bravo Murillo, 19-1'B, E-28015 Madrid, Spain*

In Italy: Please write to *Penguin Italia s.r.l., Via Felice Casati 20, I-20104 Milano*

In France: Please write to *Penguin France S.A., 17 rue Lejeune, F-31000 Toulouse*

In Japan: Please write to *Penguin Books Japan. Ishikiribashi Building, 2-5-4, Suido, Tokyo 112*

In Greece: Please write to *Penguin Hellas Ltd, dimocritou 3, GR-106 71 Athens*

In South Africa: Please write to *Longman Penguin Books Southern Africa (Pty) Ltd, Private Bag X08, Bertsham 2013*